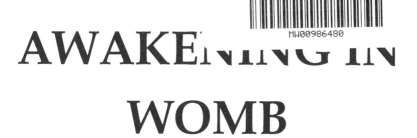

AWAKENING IN WOMB

SCIENCE OF BLUEPRINTING THE SUBCONSCIOUS MIND OF YOUR UNBORN

By
Dr Monika Singh

"Nothing is permanent, neither appreciation nor criticism; neither acceptance nor rejection."

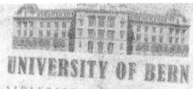

UNIVERSITY OF BERN

SIDLERSTRASSE 5 3012 BERN

06 June, 1907

Dear Mr. Einstein,

Your application for the Doctorate has not been successful at this time and as such you are not eligible for the position of Associate Professor.

While you posed an interesting theory in your article published in "Annalen der Physik", we feel that your conclusions about the nature of light and the fundamental connection between space and time are somewhat radical. Overall, we find your assumptions to be more artistic than actual Physics.

Sincerely yours,

Professor Wilhelm Heinrich, Ph.D.
Dean of Sciences

Finding Your Way Home; My Disclaimer

People often ask me if I have contact with the Masters, or the incoming New borns' consciousness. The messages come from everywhere. Some of the messages come from your own meditations and some of the information comes through feelings, at a level of understanding that It is very difficult to translate into words. For some concepts, there are no words.

Much of the knowledge comes through examples and experiences, as I have elaborately described in this book. There is a complete and a coherent spiritual philosophy in the quotes, the words, the stories and the reflections that do wonders.

Only LOVE is real. Love is the energy of incredible power and strength. We are all made of this energy.

With love, I ask you to own your POWER to imprint the sub conscious mind of your unborn child with more AWARENESS, NEUTRALITY AND RESPONSIBILITY. The content of this book is NOT a replacement to your medical Obstetric visits, but a knowledge which is your companion on your journey into parenthood. This neither is a subject of medical Obstetrics or Gynaecology. This is a volume of my inner guidance, my experiences, research, results that I have obtained with my patients who along with the contemporary medical advice took advantage of this knowledge and today are the parents of some of the most incredible children. Also of immense value are the references taken from my esteemed colleagues across the Globe who stand committed to bring about a change in the way we nurture and bring up our New Progeny...

Let's together BIRTH THE NEW EARTH...

DEDICATION

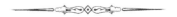

BIRTH THE NEW EARTH

I dedicate this book to the Miracle Babies, who are growing into the future. To the Miracle Babies who are yet to walk the planet. The ones who have been here in the past and have not left this world without their mark being felt.

Monika

SPIRITUALITY AND SCIENCE: ARE THEY DISTINCT?

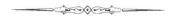

Spirituality Is The Science of Gods; Humans Can't Think of Proving It..

Spirituality is all that deals in spirit. Spirit is energy! All that is living or non-living, as per human perception and comprehension, is energy. The basic sub-atomic particles vibrate because of this energy. At the quantum level, the living and non-living quantities are the same! Similarly, all that human brain and mind have proven has become science. Whatever remains unproven by human potential is referred to as spirituality, the phenomenon being concerned with the human spirit or soul, as opposed to material or physical paraphernalia.

TO YOU, FROM ME

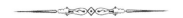

To You,

It is no coincidence that as you hold this book, you plan to be in the family way or you already are! You are about to embark on a journey which has the potential to transform you, and it is up to you to make the choice and take on this wonderful joyride, This book has been written for you, your unborn and already born. It is time for you to take a leap in your consciousness, with faith, trust, belief and hope. Let it fill you with that unconditional love which will allow the best to unfold and happen!

This book has been written with the intent to reach out to the future parents, couples with fertility issues, expecting parents, carrying mothers, the parents of newborn infants and also for the people who guide couples through the pregnancies, This book is relevant to one and all, as most of us are born with the potential to become parents or we already are! Most of the contents of this book is inner-guided and supported with the relevant research. May this book bring you immense joy, peace of mind, blessings, contentment, guidance, clarity and solutions you have been looking for.

With lots of love, good wishes and joy,
Dr. Monika Singh

FOREWORD

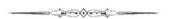

Dr. Monika Singh's book is about blueprinting love, joy, peace, and harmony right from the start...in the womb! Comprehensive, forward-thinking and a blend of science and spirituality, Awakening in Womb is a must-read for anyone who wants their child to have, not a fighting start but a loving start!

Dr. Marissa Pei, aka 'the Asian Oprah'
media personality, Life Balance coach, TV commentator,
Motivational speaker and Loving mom! California, USA

"Awakening in womb" is an enlightening journey into the programmes and patterns which blueprint a newborn life. As Dr Monika Singh explains how to call in and nurture a high vibration soul--more than old souls--she speaks of calling in the children of the Light, the ones who are meant to bring forth the New Earth. I hope she succeeds in reaching many divine mothers who have prepared their minds and bodies to blueprint these children. Her book and her efforts are a huge contribution to our Mother Earth.

~Mana, Soul Coach, Author and Ecologist, Mumbai, India.

Awakening is a gift that chooses its recipients. And what a gift to be chosen, to be an awakening facilitator in the womb! I believe this book can change the way parents view fertility and birthing and provide a guideline to all those who have a dream to raise awakened children. For years now, I have remained convinced that we are all born with a certain gift and it's with sheer hard work, perseverance and guidance that we activate our destiny. May you find here all the guidance that you need on your crucial journey!

Sidra Jafri, Awakening Facilitator and Author of the
Book, 'The Awakening -- 9 Principles for Finding
the Courage to Change Your Life'', London, U.K

Dear Monika,

Congratulations for your brilliant effort. The power to hold today and create tomorrow lies in the Energy within us. This book, ''Awakening in Womb'', not only glorifies the energy we hold, but also enlightens us about the parenthood. It describes how energy can transform the lives of unborn and newborn. It awakens the minds of the readers and remains your breath-taking achievement.

Dr Sanjay Garg,
Past President, Indian Academy of Pediatrics
I. A. P. , Uttarakhand , India.

Dr Monika writes about the Blueprint of the subconscious of the unborn. She is working with the babies in womb ! I believe in her processes completely and with the studies that I have done, in quantum physics , neurosciences and psychology, I know that the processes she is using will impact her clients and the future babies of the world in a way that we can never imagine ! These processes that she is using are from ancient wisdom something that we can all really connect to. These are the processes which will change your life and the life of your children and for the generations to come. I highly recommend that you use these processes in your life, because how you connect with your babies now, is going to make a huge difference for the rest of their lives.

Malissa Binkley, Founder Intuitive Intelligence
Academy, Florida, U.S.A

Years ago, we used to laugh it off in our night-long chit-chat sessions, but deep down in our hearts we knew she did counsel, prophesize and analyze situations to perfection, and that one day she would speak and the world would listen. This book epitomizes the person that she is. Just read and be mesmerized.

Dr Rajeev Choudhary,
Consultant Radiology and Fetal Medicine,
New Delhi, India.

Almost two decades in the field of obstetrics and fetal medicine, I always believed in the heart of my hearts that there was something working at a very different level which played a vital role in the process of conception and gestation. I saw unexplained events happening which my medical intellect just could not register, how? But when I read this book, authored by none other than my dear friend and colleague, I could feel the pieces fitting in the puzzle as she beautifully unfolds the mystery of awakening.

Dr S. Bajaj, Consultant Fetal Medicine,
Centre for Fetal Medicine, New Delhi, India

CONTENTS

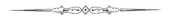

INTRODUCTION

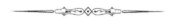

THE MOTHER, A GODDESS

A woman is just a life form until she becomes a mother, because when she carries that another soul within her body, her body becomes the Temple and she becomes the Universal Goddess.

Yes, a woman has the potential to transform into a Goddess by preparing herself to be a *Mother*. The word "MOTHER", starts with the English alphabet M, meaning *"Mercy for the other"*, where the "other" is the soul that she is carrying within.

What transforms when she becomes the medium of mercy for the other? She forgets the woman that she is. Her identities dissolve here into what she had adorned until now in her life. All she feels, thinks, nurtures and cares about now, at the core, is for the "other" or the divine soul that she carries.

Why is it that a mother is a Goddess and her body a Temple?

'Man is the Creator of God and God is the Creator of Man'

God, the universal energy, the highest power, your own higher self--you can name it whatever you resonate with-- exists and permeates through us all the living and non-living forms, at all times. The "Other Soul" too, is an energy of the Universe, the Divine. Where else would the energy of God reside, but in a Temple? And who else will have a body as a Temple, but a Goddess?

This incoming soul helps you reach out to your maximum potentials, to the deepest wells of the infinites, to unconditional love, to out-of-the-world care, to caution and protection, to be the Goddess that you are.

This unborn is a medium for any woman to undergo this highly spiritual, energetic and cosmic transformation, ie, from a woman to the 'Mother Goddess'.

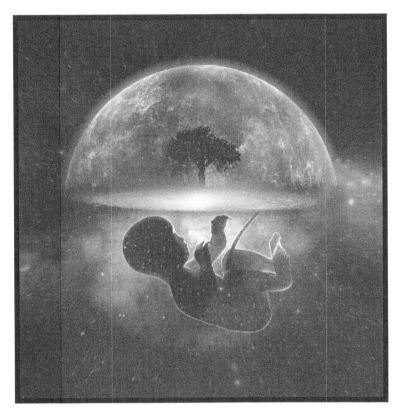

Birth The New Earth

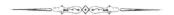

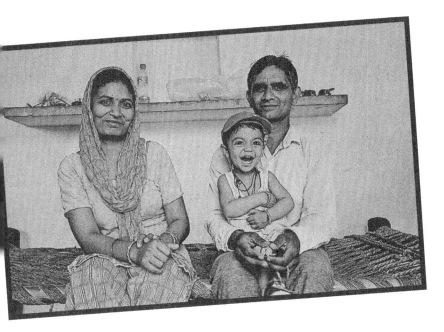

Anita and Vedpal with Krishna

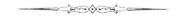

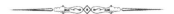

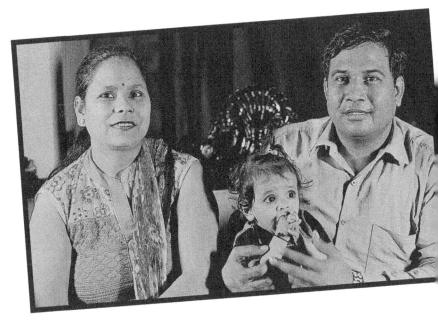

Bharti and Dharamveer with Naman

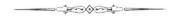

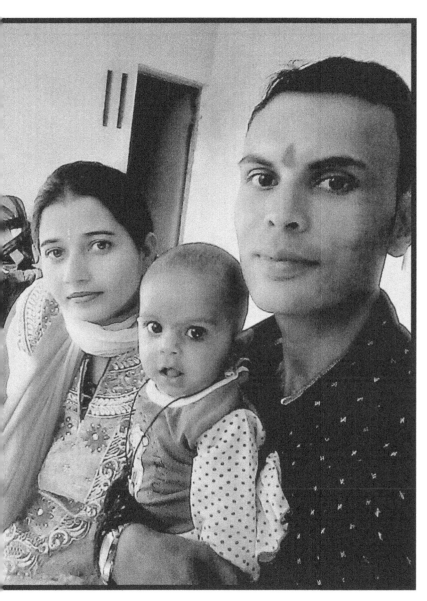

Yashodha and Gaurav with their baby girl

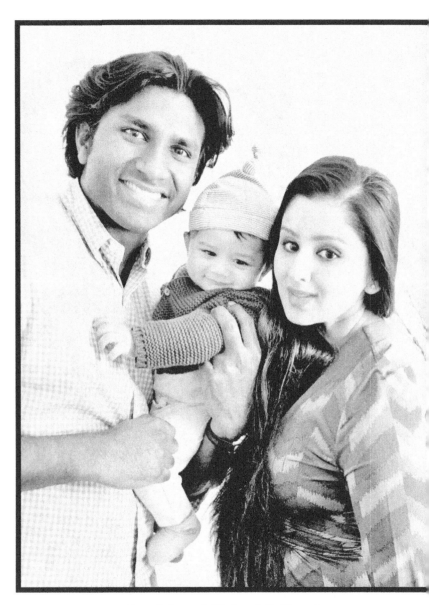

Ruchi and Tej with Ruvir

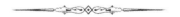

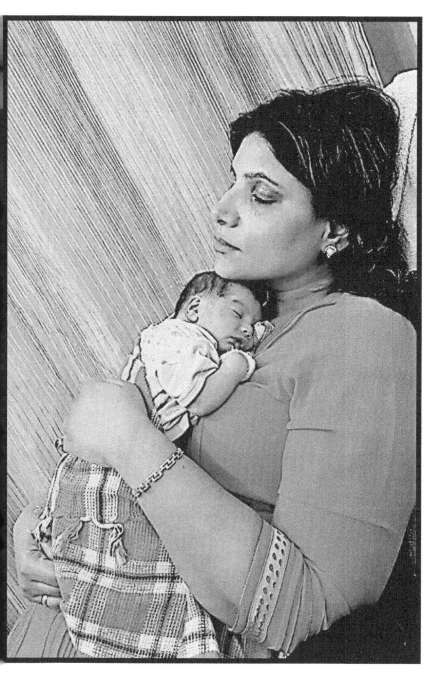

Dr. Monika Singh with one of the babies

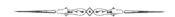

MY WAKE-UP CALL

When truth revealed itself, I acknowledged the power within.

A few years back, I came across the most profound revelation of my lifetime, the eternal truth which changed my life. The way I used to think, changed forever. I was completely transformed, not in nature, but sitting in my chair, in my study.

Today, I would like to open up my heart to you.

Not so long back ago, in 2013, over a period of few months, I had developed a strange emptiness inside me. I started feeling low (for no reason), secluded and worthless. I had a successful hospital practice, a loving, supporting and a caring husband, two beautiful children with an ever-supporting, healthy set of parents and parents-in-law. Finances were reasonably good, lifestyle was excellent , kids were growing up into amazing young people, who were achieving constantly.

In spite of everything green on the surface, something beneath shook me constantly, pulling me into a void. I would cry silently for hours, clueless, longingly, depressed, not knowing why! Pradeep, my husband, our family and friends were as clueless as I was. All were eager to do whatever they could to help me out, but no one understood anything at all. No one knew the answer to my melancholia.

But slowly, I started getting glimpses of what it could be. Someone who was deeply entrenched inside me, was breathing, living, but ignored and 'shut away', was troubling me! I was more intrigued than ever, constantly in quest of answers to my questions, inquisitiveness and the ultimate truth, searching outside of me, seeking, soaking whatever I got from anyone. I was hopping from one seminar to another, enrolling in a series of programmes and workshops. I was searching for the convincing answers from anyone and everyone, asking, asking and asking! But alas, no one had the answers!

Several books came along, one after another on the self-journey on God, science of God, on various modes of healing, karma, biographies, motivational, etc. Literary fictions, romantic novels, thrillers to which I was addicted earlier, all disappeared. I understood all these books were one's own points of wisdom and addictions. Opinions of those individuals who expressed themselves through their books and what they thought were substantive and closer to the truth of their thinking and perception.

So what was it?

Just a point of view?

Then, what about mine?

How can I know my eternal truth, my own point of view? I soon realized my truth, my point of view was inside of me, and I just had to unlock it with unflinching faith, belief and total surrender!

"No person was ever ruined from without. The final ruin comes from within..."
- Amelia Barr

I modified this quote :

"No person ever found oneself from without. The final revelation comes from within."

I had become almost a deer with soaked musk, craving for its own fragrance, running aimlessly here and there, searching outside for something that was inside me!

And I cried and cried, for tearing myself down, for doubting myself so long , living in fear of judgement.

What will people think of me?

Who am I ?

> *It may be that when we no longer know what to do, we have come to our real work.*
>
> *And then when we no longer know which way to go, we begin our real journey.*
> *--Wendell Berry*

(Poet, Cultural Critic)

I AM FAITH

You neither do live once ......nor do you die.

My essence was tied up, capped, tight and terribly strained, until I choked so much that I could explode and I did so one day.

No longer could I live the life of a blinded, pseudo jovial, external person. I needed to stop, pause, breathe, acknowledge, be tranquil and calmly go forward.

Time had come to enjoy the fragrance that looked all-pervasive and spreading.

But I had to be still, composed and non-hindring, allowing the fragrance to flow.

Convinced I stood that I was the chosen channel for this fragrance to reach out to the world. Only, I had to allow it to happen! And that was it.

And today, as I sit and write, it comes spontaneously on its own. This book comes flowing free, for I have dissolved all my identities and moved into the surrender mode.

THE ETERNITY KNOCKS, NOT ONLY ONCE..

The magic and power of subconscious revealed when subconscious revealed itself

It was a typical pleasant February of the year 2007. My life was ordinary, but adequately fulfilled. We ran a multi-speciality hospital in the western part of Delhi, having a blessed family life with our two amazing kids, aged 7+ and 5+.

The demanded care included feeding of kids, dressing them up and packing them off to school, besides my busy medical practice.

February 8, 2007: My life was to change forever..

My husband, Dr Pradeep Chauhan, a pediatrician himself, complained of a mild-fever and lethargy. He took a Paracetamol tablet and went to work. By the same evening, he was feeling more lethargic and also mildly breathless. He had his light meal, and went to rest. In the middle of the night, I saw him sitting, struggling to breathe. A little later, he was finding it difficult to lie down and breathe properly.

In the morning we sent a few blood samples to our hospital's lab. Reports revealed a mild Typhoid fever, but not severe enough to cause such breathlessness. We started the appropriate treatment, but the fever still persisted and he continued to be breathless. On walking a few steps, his condition turned still worse.

We got his detailed investigations done, including an echo, ultrasound and x-ray chest, etc,. Reports were frightening!

Pradeep had fluid filled in the membranes of all his internal organs, including liver, gall bladder, kidneys and even heart. This medical condition is called *Polyserocitis*. His heart was affected the most, leading to *pericardial effusion*. Water had filled the most of the part in between the heart and the outermost layer covering the organ, called Pericardium.

Finding the reason posed a million-dollar question.

And from here started the never-ending series of tests, trails of treatment, seeing the topmost doctors of Delhi Metropolis. All his reports were 'normal' and the treatment was just a pill of Paracetamol gulped as and when required. But the condition was not improving, the breathlessness was turning from bad to worse.

For the first time in my life, I was going through, what is called the "panicking traumatic attendant of the patient syndrome!"

Pradeep was bed-ridden, 16 days had passed, mostly on drips and on whatever treatment could be offered. We had sent the blood sample to the National Institute of Infectious Diseases, Delhi, for rigorous tests.

The reports suggested that Pradeep had infected himself with coxsakie virus, which causes influenza and cold in children, but is not fatal to them. The virus usually does not attack adults, but if it does, it comes with a highly resistant potent strain, which could cause extremely damaging, and often fatal, irreversible effects.

The treatment for this is NONE, except a supportive one.

Helplessness, despair, grief and disillusionment had overtaken the family. Pradeep was being nursed lying on his bed. I had forgotten that I had children. I was a wife first and a doctor next. I had my eyes fixed on 24 x 7, silently praying for a miracle to happen.

Hope kept us moving. That was the very reason for us to keep fighting. Lying on bed, Pradeep displayed exceptional courage and optimism and was a source of constant motivation for everyone in the family. Hiding his distressful condition, he still kept us smiling.

But my potential of rational thinking had got miserably clouded and I had become entirely non-reactive, just like a soldier going to the battle field, believing that he would be martyred..

And then arrived Feb 24, 2007, 7:40 AM

This baleful morning remains menacingly etched deep in my memory. Kids had left for school. I had just given Pradeep his Paracetamol for fever. He was sitting on his bed, my heart was skipping beats, didn't know why.

All of a sudden, he feebly pronounced my name ,"Monika"....

"I....am......slipping.....do....something......I.....am collapsing..."

Before I knew, he had collapsed, I didn't have courage to feel his pulse. I could not check his BP and I dared not to check his heart...

The doctor in me was mortally paralyzed, the wife in me was dead, the human in me was unresponsive.

Something lying deep in me surged. My soul, my entire being, as if had come alive. I took a dangling Pradeep by shoulders (don't know from where I got this strength). I was most vigorously shaking him, shouting his name, calling him 'back'. As if the entire world could hear my shrieks. People from hospital gathered hearing my cries.

I kept on calling his name endlessly, my force was getting ever stronger. I was indeed fighting a grim battle with amazing strength.

I kept on shaking him, calling his name aloud, and asking him to 'return'. I needed him, more desperately than my own life..

This went on for some 2-3 minutes that seemed to be 2-3 decades. Yet, I was fighting the fiercest battle of my life, not ready to give in.

Then , the miracle happened ! Pradeep opened his eyes and his words were:

"Why did you wake me up?.........I was going towards a beautiful blue light, through a most comforting bright tunnel of light.........I just wanted to go, why did you shout and called me back?

Then he looked all around and said, "I am fine."

No, he was not!

I immediately called cardiac ambulance and shifted him to the ICU of Escort Heart hospital.

We were still there, where we were. His pericarditis and pericardial effusion was not improving. Still, a crocin to pop in SOS and the bed rest, nothing more !

The doctors were now talking about pericardiectomy, surgical removal of the pericardium, so as to release the tightening of the heart and let it function.

I knew post this surgery Pradeep's life would be that of a vegetable. He would not be able to move beyond some 500 metres, climbing stairs would be too tedious for him and he would stay mostly indoors.

What a life would that be?

No, our dreams of a beautiful life were a way too vivid, colourful and bright. We were not ready to accept this grey, dull life. NOT THIS TIME!

We gave it a cool thought and finally requested discharge from the hospital...

We had already won a battle and, for the first time, we were not just hopeful, but positive enough to be lively and moving.

Time passed, I had made a connection with my internal self sometime back, realizing the amazing power one could have, if one wanted to!

Our lives were a gift, and we were to live. This was our second chance, to follow our true purpose, which was much beyond this regular hustle and bustle of life. If we were to live, then we had to. My inner self was guiding me and I was listening with full awareness and faith.

All these months were a life-changing, transformational time for us. We were at home, Pradeep still mostly in bed. We had gone against the surgery. Pradeep's condition was stable, but not improving. He could not climb down (if he did, it was a huge torture to his lungs. He was understandably very breathless.)

However, my connection to my inner self was getting stronger...

On that beautiful autumn day, the kids had left for their school.

8:30 AM. August last week, 2007

I intuitively stepped out of my house and went over to the district park, some 900 metres away. The morning walkers had left, a few children were playing in the park.

I sat down on one of the benches, soaking in the breeze and freshness that the morning brought and I made a phone call, the most important one which would possibly bring our lives back on the track forever.

I made a call to Pradeep and asked him to come to the park alone and take me back home. I insisted that I would not return unless he came to fetch me (He knew I wouldn't, if I said I wouldn't). I put the phone aside, my conscious brain was silent. I knew it was impossible for Pradeep to walk such a distance, but I knew something else was building up too!

I closed my eyes and prayed.

I knew he was there, when he was.

It was then, when he entered the park, put his foot on the ground inside, as I opened my eyes.

We both were warriors, but Pradeep's valiance was matchless. I sat, not excited, not jumping, not surprised, but mostly calm, as if I knew what was building up. He came close and sat beside me on the bench, put his arm around my shoulders. I leaned for his support. We were most happy, joyful, and blissful.

Pradeep was enjoying the air, the trees, and the view of greenery and colourful flowers after almost six months. We were there for over an hour.

We had tapped into the deepest secrets of the enormous power that a human mind has – the power of belief and the power of subconscious.

We walked a little in the park and went back walking. Pradeep had already walked more than 2 kilometres and climbed up stairs and had a hearty breakfast after a long time. We decided to come back to the park each day together. That was the extent of astonishing confidence that an ailing Pradeep exhibited.

By the end of September, 2007, Pradeep was walking 17 kilometres daily. His breathlessness was gone, he had shed a lot of weight and he looked 10 years younger, more active, handsome than ever.

His blood reports were normal and his pericardial effusion had gone, his heart was functioning normal, no fluid anywhere. The doctors were surprised and called it a 'miracle'.

Eventually, we knew that we had tapped into the power of the subconscious mind and had simply played around our belief system.

Every human mind carries this immense power of beliefs and subconscious. High time we took the ownership of our own belief systems and empowered ourselves with this superpower called,

Power of the Subconscious Mind

We got ourselves rid of all the medical reports, medicines, labs reports, re-did our house and completely changed track of our lives. We decided to live a life aimed at our true purpose.

It was then we decided to shut our hospital in Delhi for good and shift our base to the interior of the country's rural India, where there were no qualified doctors or medical facilities.

This place is called Chhutmalpur, 40 kms to the south of Dehradun, in the state of Uttar Pradesh, North India.

THE REVELATION

Eternity, progeny, life cycles, death, birth, all happen and have grown from a single point, a single moment, a sacred union.

And this sacred moment holds the energy of entire "beingness", and the entireness. It is the basic code which unfolds, no matter what, when, how, but unfolds; it simply does.

Being a doctor dealing with fertilization, pregnancy and childbirth, I observed that conception was involuntary and it happened at the subconscious level. One could postpone a conception through contraceptives (which fail anyways when conception has to happen !) and when it happens , it does at most unexpected times, landing mostly as a surprise or a shock !

For any conception is a cosmic conception..

The meeting point of cosmic energies is the unison. The result of the unison is also a cosmic energy, totally 'invite-able', controllable and changeable. To put it in just one phrase--this is the essence because of which, we are, who we are – the unique human beings. It does scare a bit when you come to know of your power to attract your child. This is a huge responsibility. Is not it ? How about turning this power, yet a responsibility, into an opportunity?

A human being in Hindi is *manas*, meaning *mann se*, i.e, a being who has mind, feelings and emotions. Feelings are the language of your soul. You, with your consciousness involved, consciously have the power to realize and invite this cosmic unison with another cosmic energy of the highest order.

You may do this consciously, or it may happen by default, depending upon the situations, feelings, emotions and consciousness at that moment. Hence, you end up attracting, creating and crafting the cosmic energy , your children, reflecting you and your energetic vibration that you carry!

What, if you knew, how to attract these highly evolved souls in your lives as your baby?

What, if you knew, what to do and what not to, to not attract who you don't intend to?

A POWERFUL STORY

Anita and Vedpal
(Muzaffarnagar, U.P, India)

One of days in the month of June, a slim, apprehensive, medium-height woman walked into my chamber, with eyes full of questions and yet full of hope.

I was in the middle of my busy OPD, but something about her caught my attention and made me stop. The couple had been married for nine years and never had any child. The medical reports were all normal (as per our medical perspective), her cycles were regular and healthy. Her husband had weird sperm count; sometimes sub-normal, sometimes scanty and sometimes just adequate.

The tubes were healthy, so was the anatomy and physiology of the mother's reproductive system. We did what we could do as doctors. The entire medical support, including four cycles of IUI (Intra uterine insemination), had failed. She would ovulate (have a good mature egg), but the conception would not happen!

Intuitively I knew that this was not happening and that its root lay elsewhere.

We did a few counselling sessions, did her energy clearance, helped her restore and restructure her belief and came up with the following affirmation for her (in Hindi language) :

"Hey Bhagwan, aapne mujhe itna sundar, swasth aur poore samay ka bachcha diya hai, iske liye aapka lakh-lakh dhanyawaad."

(English version: *"Thank God, you have given me this beautiful, healthy and a full-term baby, I thank you a million times for this."*)

I asked her to repeat this affirmation round the clock, visualizing a beautiful baby in her arms.

The couple did this with full faith, belief and devotion. All the medical treatment was stopped for the time being and left the rest for the energies to play. In her case, the medicines were discontinued as she had remained overloaded with medication for years and needed a break. This is done in specific cases. I would not recommend you to stop your medical treatment without a professional consultation.

I, with my skepticism and Anita gone, forgot everything and returned conveniently to my life in the whirlpool of my medical activity.

After a period of four months, Anita returned. As she sat in my chamber, my mind raced with the thoughts of recycles of IUI's and the tedious medical treatment with often negative results. I was inquisitive, but a little apprehensive too, about how she would open up on her case. Mustering a little courage, I asked her about her wellbeing.

Her face was glowing, resplendent with a divine smile. She told me that she had had check-up and that she was pregnant!

But how? I asked.

"That mantra you gave me, we chanted day and night. Just that did a miracle"

Everything came rushing back to my head and I said to myself, "Oh, so this worked with her...good!" My conviction and the ever-chasing doubts started playing games in my head. My scientific, logical mind saw it as a mere coincidence, but my deep feelings embedded in my heart knew it was the firm belief that had worked a miracle at an energetic level, to which the couple had surrendered with complete faith!

Anita gave birth to a beautiful, calm and healthy baby boy nine months after. He is called Krishna.. ☺

This was another knock of the "power of belief" in my life.

PROLOGUE

There is no knowledge which has not pre-existed, we access it—when we are ready. It has always been about discovering, re-discovering and discovering the invention.

There are many messages and revelations in this book, which are for the would-be parents, aspiring couples, and practically all who are interested in the positive growth of themselves and fellow humans in general. As a practitioner of obstetrics for about 19 years now, I have been, like so many other doctors, strongly intuitive about my patients, their diseases and outcomes.

I started "blueprinting" the babies by default long back when I was practicing at our hospital in Delhi. It was my habit to spend my own special moments with the baby that I had delivered, by talking to him/her, giving my pure love, blessings and assuring the babies with security, peace and joy.

I was surprised when their parents came back and reported as to how courageous, intelligent and loving these children were and often said, "*This baby has your stamp*" on him/her.

I used to be astonished, until 4 years ago, when I realized that I could communicate with the unborn and the newborn.

I knew we were a logical-thinking, proof-seeking, skeptical society, of which I was also a part. Self-doubt crippled me, my over-analytical, logical brain always banged me with questions like : How come? Why me? Is it possible? Or, am I just hallucinating?

But my logical mind took it too when the unborn, the fetus, had communicated with me energetically and the same came to me also through the mother later. I just smiled, conveying : "I already know this!"

As I grew restless, resisting and questioning myself too often, my connection grew stronger. Soon, I was on a journey of self-acceptance with humility and surrender. Soon, my logical mind got satisfied with thousands of cases standing in testimony, proving and realizing that these were the *"gifts"* from a doctor through the beneficence of higher powers. It is said, "With realization, comes responsibility". I realized and reminded myself that I was nobody and yet everybody. What came to me was not mine ; it was just coming *through me!*

I started having visions after visions and started waking up at 4:30 AM daily without an alarm bell to wake me up, as if someone was poking and asking me to wake up. It was just "the calling" that woke me up!

I started breathing completely in the vibrations of gratitude, thanking the universe for choosing me as it's instrument for carrying out the healing work on mothers, fathers and the unborns. The communications became stronger and I was soon talking to the unborns as early as at the end of the 12th week.

I would be communicating, through the baby, about the mother's emotional and mental state, what it was doing to the unborn and the willingness, force, enthusiasm of the unborn to come to this world. Sometimes, the baby at 28 weeks would communicate the desire to go back and leave the body of the mother, as the mother was resisting, not willing to change her attitude and her vibrations which were to be alleviated through this pregnancy. In such cases, in extreme conditions, the baby would even want to leave, no more desiring to come to this world through this mother. Such a pregnancy ran into difficult and challenging situations, inviting fetal and maternal diseases, quite often leading to "intra uterine death" or IUD, as it is called.

You, as the mother and the father, are the ones to decide your baby's fate and future, through the choices you are making and the decisions that you are taking.

Remember BABA, a commonly used word in different contexts to be a reminder of 'be aware, be awake'

By being fully conscious of your environment, your own state of being, your thoughts and your beliefs, you can easily craft and help your baby be the highest that it could be.

LEVELS OF MIND

There are four levels of consciousness in four areas each of any human being. These are the areas of body (physical), emotional, mental and spiritual. The four levels of consciousness are conscious mind, subconscious mind, unconscious mind and the super conscious mind. All four are applicable in the same way to all four different bodies(we shall ponder over these four bodies later in the book).

The conscious mind is to actively complete a task. For example, if you needed to visit someone, you would have to move out of your home, travel, meet that person and have a conversation. This is accomplished with the conscious and a little with the subconscious mind.

The unconscious mind is the automatic part—it regulates your body temperature, keeps your heart pumping and performs all the automated tasks that keep you alive. There are also other actions that can be developed with conscious practice. Wim Hof, also called the Ice Man, is known to consciously regulate and control his body temperature in ice and regulate his immune system.

The subconscious mind is like a storage box of all the information. If one has no brain damage, then one can always dive into the information stored in and make the best of the inner knowledge. One of the better methods of retrieving information is hypnosis, or the deep sleep, but it can also be accessed through the lucid dreams and self-hypnosis. The subconscious mind has a super computer style of being able to access information. Let's say you attended a party, your subconscious mind will always store all the figures and names of the people present there which otherwise we always forget. Not only that, it will store also every item of clothes worn by a person. Every aspect of the night you viewed will be tucked away in your little super computer. Your subconscious mind is the warehouse of all visual, tactile, olfactory, sensory, gustatory (for taste), mental, emotional, physical information your mind has stored from the inference of your experiences.

A basic, repetitive inflow of the information becomes a conditioned habit, and hence your belief system. Let's take this simple example of your birth. When you were born, you were not aware of the existance of two sexes, but as you were told about your sex, it became your belief and hence your truth! Similarly, approximately 30,000 thoughts are generated in an average human mind every day, as is frequently stated by Dr Deepak Chopra, M.D, a big name in the field of spirituality and wellness. The repetitive ones become your beliefs and the truths of life. A large part of these belief systems are programmed while the baby is still inside the mom's body. This happens as a result of the mother's experiences.

The subconscious mind is strictly habitual and doesn't know good, bad, right or wrong. It just has the information and the stored belief patterns, on the basis of which the life unfolds! The frequency of the energetic vibration of the corresponding information and the belief becomes the source of external manifestation in your physical reality. This is how the "Law of Attraction" works.

"Our physical manifestation is not what we desire, it is who we are..."

A consciously programmed subconscious mind of your unborn will lead to the formation of serving believes and truths of the life of the unborn. Let the truths be full of unconditional love, courage, kindness, peace and neutrality!

Lastly, you have your super conscious mind. This is when you act in an the automatic way at the four levels, one may call this state that of FLOW. Sometimes it shows itself in glimpses, lasting for a very short span and sometimes the entire life is spent in it. It is like being guided by a higher power. Once you are aligned with your true purpose in life, you are at the super conscious level. Call this the level of FLOW.

OUR OWN LEVELS OF EXISTENCE

On your individual and collective journey towards peace and enlightenment, you are challenged at different levels for different emotions and understandings. Become aware that these emotions propel you to stride up and forward. You could be stuck at anyone of it, getting out of this stuck loop could take an entire lifetime, one moment or just a fraction of a second to change that vibration.

Your entire life can run on a single pattern or emotion. You can go on and on and get stuck in a viscous loop of Karma with different people—living or dead, with vows, promises, curses and patterns of give-and-take or of the karma.

Becoming aware of these thought patterns, blockage patterns and repeating patterns is essential for the shift and the change of the orbit, i.e., the change in your thought patterns and emotions that you are stuck in.

The belief of existence from the perspective of the level of consciousness, right from the frequency of shame, 20 hertz to that of enlightenment 700+hertz, *(refer to the levels of consciousness)*, is not a linear, up moving, upgrading graph of all frequencies, in fact it is, one or more or most of them, existing together, and this co-existence of different energies forms a unique human energetic existence, and what we show up with, is our most dominant frequency of vibration.

The permutation and combination of these different vibrations with respect to intensity, frequency of experience, intention for awareness, intensity of karmic bonds, karma, vows, contracts, curses, etc, make up a unique human energetic flux, culminating into our entire physical existence in wholeness, formulating a Human Energetic System, i.e., A Human Being, meaning YOU!

This energetic system is translated into pure *"beingness"*, something that is highly variable, changeable and changes constantly and, thus, remains highly adaptive.

- The *"POWER"* is to be able to identify the energetic pattern, to break stagnation and repetition of similar patterns through the lifetime with different people. This pregnancy is a medium of accelerating your vibrational switch, energetic enhancement towards faith and unconditional love. The equation has changed a bit though, the time has come for you to evolve, you may do so and become eligible to attract that higher vibrating soul in your life, who is not only for you, but for the betterment of our human race!

- Yes, it is possible!

Earlier, it was 'birth to evolve', now it is shifting to 'evolve to birth'.

Before you were conceived,
I wanted you.
Before you were born,
I loved you.
Before you were here an hour
I would die for you.
This is the miracle of life.

- Maureen Hawkins

"How people treat you is their karma,
How you react is yours..."
Wyne W. Dyer

KARMA AND CLEARANCE

Karma and the karmic patterns is the game of execution and action. It is based on our belief patterns, our thought forms and the information we have stored in our system, in our body about our behaviors and reactions to the actions of other people and vice versa. This leads to give-and-take account keeping. The reflection of our life is a cumulative 'effect' of the 'cause' we experience. Playing the game, we may stay in a karmic loop forever, held up in a karmic cycle with a person or a different set of people at a certain vibrational field. When you find the entire cycle repeating, you start feeling frustrated and claustrophobic, you saturate yourself and this leads to further deterioration.

With awareness and intention, one can shift his or her mind-set and thought patterns. One can pull oneself out of this entire vibrational existence and jump to another set of vibrations. Here, of course, it shall be another set of karmas waiting and if this vibration is that of love, then what you manifest, reciprocate and experience shall be love.

Again, it is a *choice*, as it is always!

Mostly, difficulty in conception is due to the blockages often at the root level, the basic existence and the survival level.

We tend to cocoon and defend ourselves when we get threatened at any level—energetic, physical, mental or emotional. As we react in the form of outbursts, outrages and explanations, we quickly commence a defence mechanism of shielding/cocooning ourselves, by erecting that impermeable wall of defence. This shield wall could be in the form of curses, vows, or even through simple assertions, 'self-promises', such as, 'I will never...,' or 'I will forever..' With the intention of punishing others, we forget that when we intend to punish others, we punish ourselves too.

Here are a few examples of very innocently made remarks, but with an intensity to punish someone like : "I will not bear the child to this family", or out of the fear of having witnessed a death or a tragedy during the birthing process, or having been through a traumatic childhood, when either of your parents had to suffer raising you and your siblings – your thought, 'my mother would have been so good, all by herself, if only she didn't have us as her kids'(without actually ever asking her if it was true. All presumptions! On the contrary, maybe, you the kids were the driving force of her life!).

These remarks, thought forms, are simple promises and often one-liners spoken to self. They remain in our subconscious mind for a long time and these belief patterns are the ones which run the show of our lives.

It is not necessary to go through the entire cycle of karmic experience and resolution. The karmic pattern, the karma, can be deleted/ its intensity reduced, in a simple statement like :

"I declare my karma complete with so and so across all timelines, space and dimensions".

This declaration is widely used by intuitive guides and healers.

Maybe, you will not fully delete your karma (though there is a high possibility that you will, once you learn how to reach the deepest layers of your subconscious mind). You are capable enough to resolve the karma. All you need to do is to learn and integrate. If need be, just be prepared to attract another person, who will pose a similar challenge. As you identify your own pattern and make a choice to consciously learn and integrate from that lesson, you already have shifted your vibrational frequency in that very moment.

There is no rocket science to awakening; only awareness, integration and actions are the keys.

Once you realize your truth and open up to yourself, all your knots and blockages open up and you start receiving the channels of blessings and guidance, which, in fact, were always flowing. This is the state of BLISS or super consciousness.

SONI'S STORY

Soni, a young girl with regular cycles and a fit body in the fourth year of her marriage, was still not able to conceive. She had a history of recurring endometriotic cysts, both blood filled. Each time she went to the doctor, her cysts were diagnosed. She underwent several hormonal treatments, and her cysts would go only to come back repeatedly.

When she came to me, I sensed that there was a deeper cause, which was buried deep inside her subconscious mind. Upon a probing session, it was found that as a child, she had witnessed her aunt undergo the agony and suffering of not being able to conceive a baby all her life, and lived a life of shame, guilt and misery. She unknowingly had made a belief that infertility is the worst thing to happen, and she will not let this misery touch her. The subconscious mind understands the gravity and the major words. It registered the word infertility most strongly. Also, to undergo the experience of faith and surrender, she had to experience difficult and challenging fertility issues.

"Infertility", "not conceiving child", "misery", and "agony" were her prime words and she had formed a solid belief and her subconscious mind was programmed on infertility and she promptly landed into it.

We took up her case both at contemporary medical and energetic levels and did her subconscious mind reprogramming. Not only did her cysts resolve spontaneously over a short period of time, but also did she conceive spontaneously and later gave birth to a healthy baby girl.

Miracle!

Really?

There are several energy disturbances that need to be corrected to have a fit and blissful physical state of being. As Sidra Jafri says, "Energy is everything and everything is energy" If diving into this world of energy, equip yourself well (with unconditional love, calmness and peace), and then play the game hard, and only you shall win.

PART 1

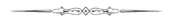

THE COSMIC CONCEPTION

THE IDEAL TIME

The time before the three months of conception is the crucial time of your pregnancy.

The period carries in itself the blueprint of conception, the blueprint of three trimesters--the blueprint of the health of mother and of baby, and to an extent, the blueprint of the birthing process too. This means the three months, prior to the conception, cannot, at any cost, be overlooked anytime.

When you are planning to have a baby, act of culmination should be performed at the night time, hours leading to the midnight, and certainly not at the day time.

During the three months (ideal) prior to the conception, there should be:

1. **No Aggression:** The aggression stays for weeks to months to years (on an average 2 to 3 weeks, actively) energetically in your electromagnetic field. When the incoming soul passes ,through this field inside you, it carries this energy if not cleansed already, infusing it with itself. Staying in the state of aggression during the crucial nine months, you cause severe damage not only to yourselves, but also to your ongoing pregnancy. This may invite a lot of obstetric and birthing problems, beside several future challenges to your child.

2. **Happiness Is Needed** between the couple. A happy aura is an inviting aura for a soul of a higher vibration. More peaceful, more blissful, more awakened and a much more happy soul is attracted to this couple and embraces the

developing body inside the mother's womb. The pregnancy and delivery are both uneventful. This family rises to two levels higher just by bringing this soul home.

3. **No fear or doubt:** The fears and doubts have to be de-rooted from very deep energies, from the basic quantum levels, through procedures and techniques and they may be replaced with courage assurance and confidence. These fears and doubts have a deeper effect on the babies , such children may grow up with low self-esteem, low self-worth, jealousy and timidity, just to name a few.

4. **Unconditional love, Courage and Confidence:** When the conception happens at this vibration, the kid lives in the energy of power victor and not in victim consciousness. Faith engulfs them and because of this faith, these children remain subconsciously aware of the power of surrender. Further in their lives, they attract abundance, remain very courageous and live blissful lives.

   These individuals are also bestowed with an exceptional power of *healing. They are truthful, integrated, highly intuitive, aligned to their soul's purpose and do not deviate easily.* These children are *peaceful, flexible, understanding, out-of -the-box thinkers with high IQ, EQ and SQ.* They have a massive capacity and potential to become country/ world leaders.

5. **No Guilt:** It is the lowest emotion on the level of consciousness, lower than anger, fear, pride and justification. Here the person/couple lives in the gross, very heavy state of disempowering beliefs. Such mothers could be diabetic, hypertensive, epileptic or suffering from

some other chronic/major diseases. They also attract babies who have tendencies to be depressed, sad, unhealthy and are prone to remaining sick individuals when grown up. Such kids have frequent visits to doctors with acute and chronic ailments, such as asthma, allergies breathing issues, heart problems which are commonly associated with guilt. A major work needs to be done to get rid of it energetically, replacing it with confidence, freedom and self-love.

6. **State of Love:** It is the basic frequency of this realm, i.e., our planet. It is also the key to all abundance, happiness, bliss, 'moksha', 'nirvana', contentment, love, wealth, energy, and whatever positives one could possibly imagine. Here, the baby is highly aligned to its soul's purpose, is generally extremely loving and caring with high EQ and IQ. Such a genius may have the potential to be a scientist or a celebrity researcher. These babies grow up to become world leaders, spiritual gurus, top businessmen and have highly philosophical minds. They share their wisdom and knowledge with the world from the very early stages of their lives.

COSMIC CONCEPTION: A REMINDER

1. It will be better if coitus is performed at night.
2. All previous unwanted energies should be removed, cleared and replaced with the needed ones.
3. Should be performed with patience, love, ease and grace, absorbing completely in each other's energies and giving in completely to each other with no inhibition.
4. Both partners may experience bliss together.

5. Both of them should be together for some time, after the coitus has taken place.

6. The mother decides when to let go of her husband/partner.

7. She may get up and have bath at around 4.45 AM, 5.00 AM, if possible.

8. Both should pray for gratitude and positive affirmation, regarding the soul's attraction.

9. If even after following this, result doesn't flow in, regular affirmation, deep meditation and patience will show you the way.

THE ENERGETIC PROCESS

Attracting A Higher Order Soul

It is no coincidence that you are reading this process because you have the potential to attract the soul of higher order. So, just let go of all the doubts, embrace belief completely and follow this process with faith and surrender.

After setting your intention to conceive and attract a high vibrational soul into your life, you have to make a conscious effort to raise your own vibrations, so as to be able to sustain these very high, beautiful vibrations of the unborn.

Start by repeating to yourself and declaring to the universe:

I invite, allow and accept the highest vibrational energy being to bless us and our lives and the lives of several others on this planet, by choosing us as his/ her parents for re-incarnating for this lifetime. Thank you.

After the intention and invitation, it is time to indulge in the sacred act of oneness. It is highly advisable and recommended to follow this energetic invitation process—for the higher being to choose you and your partner as its parents, if aligned!

Prior to this, you must be off any alcohol and non-vegetarian food for at least a period of 45 days, (3 months is ideal for both partners).

Please find an audio-directed process at *www.birththenewearth.com*

After waking up between 3:50 and 4:00 am, (4: 00 am is the ideal time.) both of you sit east-facing, in the north-east direction of your house. If this is not possible, you may sit on the terrace or even the balcony of your house facing eastwards. The female sits on the right side of her husband, holding hands, the man's right hand palm facing upwards and the female's left palm on his.

Close your eyes and start inhaling through your nostrils and exhaling through your mouth. The exhalation is longer than the inhalation. Let any interfering thoughts come and pass, just focus on your breathing. Visualize your true self as a shining pointed dot in the centre of your forehead, the bright light radiating out of it and spreading throughout your body, soaking each and every cell of it in its rich, blissful, calming energies. It is now expanding to the outside of you, surrounding and soaking your partner in it completely, a homogeneous submersion of both of you in the expanded source energy of you both.

Visualize another shining dot, a soothing, serene relaxing energy descending upon you both and entering the combined source energetic field of you both. This energy is circulating around you in the clockwise direction, spinning on its own and while revolving it is getting dissolved in the energies of you both. (Just like the sugar crystal gets dissolved while being stirred in water or milk) This is the powerful source energy of you three.

Now visualize the entire energetic matrix surrounding you both, entering your (female's) body completely surrounding her from all directions being sucked inside from her heart centre (bright shiny green in colour). From here, this powerful, love-filled energy is entering your bright, shiny, yellow-coloured solar plexus centre (just above the naval). From here, it is further descending down to the sacral plexus, the centre for creation, descending lower down just above the pubic bone, bright shining expansive orange colour, from here, this vibrant energy is entering the reproductive organs and the uterus, welcome it into your physical, mental, emotional and energetic bodies, your existing energetic life system.

Thank God and be in gratitude to the higher power, higher self, cosmic light, whichever source energy you resonate with most, for allowing this precious moment to be a part of your experience.

Continue to stay in the ecstatic moment. When you feel comfortable, open your eyes and hydrate yourself. You may repeat this as often as you want, baring day 4, 9, and 14th in the lunar cycles of both waxing and whining phases of moon.

REPEAT: *"Thank you Almighty, for this high vibrational soul in our lives as our unborn child. Thank you for this divine pregnancy and a beautiful healthy baby at the time of its birth and after".*

BLOCKAGE IN CONCEPTION: KARMA PERHAPS?

Sometimes there could be a family karmic block, which is prevailing. If your siblings, cousins, uncles and aunts also have cases of fertility issues, then this is a case of family karmic block and has to be resolved at the family level, with awareness, intention and integration of all the family members. The cumulative, synchronized energy will find its way in.

Till the time the energy of insecurity and negativity is in the auric field , these mental blocks, promises, or unserving beliefs continue to persist which may be cleared and replaced with much ease. Once the experiences become intense, they start taking shape in the body in the form of discomforts, problems, aches, pains and diseases. The females start manifesting irregular, fluctuating menstrual cycles, cysts, fibroids, menstrual disorders and various hormonal imbalances.

All this leads to our getting stuck in the vicious cycle of "karma" and sabotages.

KARMIC CYCLE:

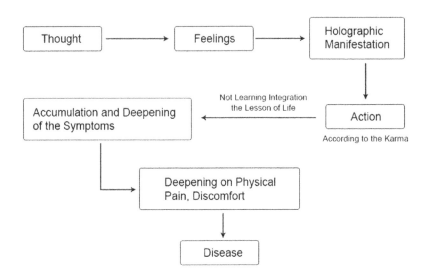

THE CYLE OF KARMA

AND GETTING OUT OF IT

The vicious karmic cycles and karmic patterns may continue for many lifetimes, one lifetime, decades, years, months, weeks, days, or a few seconds . Time is relative and exists for us proportional to our own experiences.

The essence of the vicious cycle is to let us be aware of our lessons and integrate it. All is present in the NOW. *"Everything Is Present Only and Exclusively In the Now"*. Time is only mind-conceived : the mind gets us into the never-ending, infinite seeming loops of karmic patterns and time frames. It is to be understood and felt that what may take a life time for one to understand and integrate, could take a little or no time for another.

Getting out of the karmic pattern comes down to a very simple yet *profound* phenomenon, called **Choice.**

The time moves from moment to moment with choice to choice. Our entire journey of life is an affect of choices that we have made and are still making. The entire cycle of karma, the illusion, the 'MAYA', is addictive as it includes a lot of juicy drama inclusive of juicy addictive emotions of pain, hurt, fear, guilt, grief, shame, anger and remorse. These emotions are strong enough vibrational energies to keep us attached and addicted to them.

Getting out of this vicious, addictive cycle of illusion would need one single thing—THE CHOICE, to get out!

Eligibility of coming out of this vicious cycle would take two things primarily:

The **awareness** and the **choice** period!

Yes, it is that simple, as all great things are very simple and easily available. Similarly, breaking of the karmic pattern requires becoming aware and making a choice of getting out of it.

And then this choice has to be put into action. Keep calm, believe that this is simple and applicable and welcome to the world of change and transformation of destinies.

The Creator has given His power in your hands to create his own children. The only thing now left is to acknowledge your power and embrace it with awareness and intention and execute it in the best possible way.

Very simple, isn't it?

Let me explain this in the next chapter.

'ONLY' POSITIVE THINKING IS CRIPPLING !

The awareness now is here and the choice too stands right there. The distance between making a choice and executing it could be vast, perhaps the time of one's entire lifespan.

Here comes the part play of our incredibly powerful minds. My own life's experiences and several path-breaking researches, including one on cells by Dr Bruce Lipton, provide insights into how the body-mind-spirit pathways work.

I do not believe that simply harbouring positive thoughts always leads to physical changes. You need more than just "positive thinking" to harness control of your body and your life. In spite of daily readings of positive quotes, social media circulating messages, blogs and several positive-thinking self-help books, the change does not happen.

Why?

The answer is simple!

What people don't understand is the seemingly singular and separate subdivisions of mind—the conscious and subconscious minds are interdependent. The conscious mind is the creative one that easily absorbs the positive thoughts. In contrast, the subconscious mind is a warehouse of collected belief patterns, conditionings and action patterns which have formed mainly through the blueprinting done during the golden time of pregnancy. This depends upon the experiences and blueprints of one's own parents and families and our experiences which lead to the stimulus – response mechanism. Subconscious mind is strictly habitual. It will keep on playing the same behavioural responses to life's signals over and over again.

It is now a proven fact that subconscious mind is billions of times stronger than the conscious mind. You may repeat the positive affirmations time and again, like reciting ever day that your pancreas is getting stronger and repaired, but this doesn't lead to positive results in the physical manifestations. The belief pattern that money is difficult to earn is programmed in the childhood just too easily. Similarly, the programme that the normal deliveries have become rare and caesareans are becoming more common is running your life's manifestations. What do you think this is going to manifest? A caesarean and lack of money, of course!

The techniques of re-programming the subconscious mind are easy, learnable and applicable.

Once you have made a choice to replace your identified, unserving pattern, you have accomplished it by 50%. The rest 50% shall be achieved by believing the choices to be real and living the life created out of that choice, even if it is done consciously for sometime in the beginning. In fact, your mind will believe what you want it to believe.

GETTING OUT OF THE KARMIC LOOP

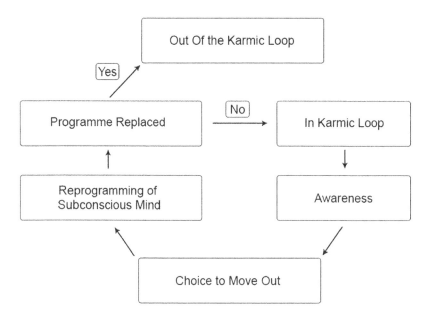

THE THREE 'GUNAS'

The Eligibility to attract, invite and allow the higher soul through yourself

All of us have these three basic tendencies—the nature of the creative force in our energy system. The force of the creative energy comprises three fundamental principles or attributes, called the "*gunas*" in Sanskrit, meaning tendencies.

- *Sattva*
- *Rajas*
- *Tamas*

Satva is the principal of purity, *Rajas* is the principal of activity and *Tamas* is the principal of inertia (inaction). It is the dominance of these tendencies that determines the innate nature of any human being. At the level of the mind, the attributes imparted by *SATTVAGUNA* are clarity, alertness, alacrity, sensitivity, purity, kindness, helpfulness, spirit of team work and contentment. The dominant trait of the people with this 'guna' is calmness. They stay in the present and have a presence of peace surrounding them. They have excellent memories.

'RAJOGUNA' revolves around the ego, the 'I'. Egotism is the prime feature of *Rajoguna*. Such a person is not a team player, he thinks that he is the best, and he knows the best. Such people are restless and anxious, apprehensive about what others say about them. They are mostly concerned about their recognition, being heard and liked. People with dominant *Rajoguna* are rash and bash, give in to impulsive, impetuous behaviour and often land hurting themselves and others. These people do not give time for the formation of the memory, for their mind is always moving from A to D to E to Z at a breakneck speed. They are forgetful and lose track of direction.

"*TAMOGUNA*" literally means darkness. The entire world of objects, including the body emanates from '*tamoguna*'. People with *tamoguni* tendencies do not feel like doing anything, they are apathetic, lack enthusiasm, are pessimists, have recurring bouts of depression and are prone to despondency. These people cry at the drop of the hat. Anger is another sign of *tamoguna*. A *Satvaguni* person, on the other hand, will utilize anger for specific purposes.

A person is always a combination of these three gunas. What matters the most is the proportion of the three and the dominant trait.

For example, a *tamsik* mother will thrash her misbehaving child, and then hurt herself for having produced such a brat. A *rajasik* mother may as well beat up her child, but stops at that. But a *sattvik* mother will neither whip the child nor herself, she will analyze the child's behaviour and get to the root of it. She will get a solution and explain it to the youngster in an appropriate manner. (See insights in the book, *Mind Undressed*, by Anandmurti Guruma)

The proportion and balance of these *gunas* make us who we are. If we are eligible to attract that *Highly Evolved Being* (HEB) in our life in the form of our child, we need to qualify and be eligible for it.

Your *sattvik guna*, must be raised up to 50%. There are various ways to achieve it, and remember, you cannot force the tendencies to change as they are inherent at the basic level, but with a conscious effort and awareness, it is possible and achievable. Are you willing to raise your consciousness and be ready and available?

With *'gunas'* as the reference point, when we talk about our physical bodies, 50% has to be *tamas* always, as it consists of the dense parts--the bones, muscles, cartilage organs and the organ systems. The rest is water (*rajas*) and air, fire and space (*sattva*). You cannot exist without *tamas*, i.e, your physical body. However, you can cautiously balance the *rajas* and *sattva* contents. When the *tamas* is raised beyond 50% in the physical existence of the body, the *sattva* guna falls.

While talking of these gunas for our mental and emotional bodies, the *sattva* guna can be raised to any extent, depending on your wish (generally not beyond a 70%, as you still have to live in this world of surviving reality, be a part of it), but when the *sattva* guna falls down beyond 40% in our mental, and emotional bodies, our existing life becomes heavier, full of obstructing challenges, fear, anger, suppression, dominance, feeling of a caged prisoner. If you are feeling heavy, not cheerful at this given moment, step back and review your life in the context to gunas. You have the ability to increase your *sattvik* guna in your existence, the *tamsik* and the *rajsik* gunas will automatically fall in proportion.

WAYS TO RAISE YOUR SATTVIK GUNA

Go to bed early and rise early
Avoid night work, especially in the hours leading to midnight as this period is *tamsik*. Even biologically, the human body is not designed for any kind of nocturnal work.

Morning hours are full of *sattva*, when awake during those hours, we naturally absorb the positive energy. The time period, called *Brahma Muhurata*, which begins 90 minutes before sunrise and ends at sunrise, is especially potent with high *sattvik* cosmic vibrations.

Meditate
The early morning hours are ideal for meditation. Meditation could be simply focusing on your breath, aiming to achieve the condition of thoughtlessness. When you are thoughtless, you become completely and fully present in the moment 'NOW'. This moment of an 'empty now' could be the longest, deepest and the most fulfilling moment of your lifetime. This moment gives you an opportunity to find your life's true purpose and find the path to reach your highest potential in quest of fulfilling the purpose of your life.

Spend Lonely Hours with Yourself and Nature
Nature and connecting with Mother Earth have a deep positive effect on the mind. Spend some time alone with yourself and Mother Nature and allow her to nurture you in solitude. Talk to yourself aloud. Who but you would understand you the most and best? This also helps in your own inner connection and deeper journey within yourself.

Regulate Your Sex Life, Avoid Gambling and Stay Clear of Intoxicants

Sex is a *rajsik* activity. It is the most powerful energy of pull and push, the energy of creativity. Too much of indulgence in mechanical sex can be limiting and encaging. A balanced, high-energy, love-filled sex can be liberating. Beware of multiple partner relationships and physical associations. This could lead to unnecessary chaos and energetic confusion, manifested in anxiety, turmoil and fear in your life, thus raising your *tamsik* tendencies. Addictions to physically abusive substances, alcohol and drugs have a huge potential to raise your *tamsik* vibrations.

Spend Time Away From Technology

Technology is *rajsik* in nature. It infuses us with an attitude of controllership and information technology is all the more *tamoguna*. It makes our mind restless, anxious and comparative. Strictly stay away from technology during meditation and when you are spending time alone with nature.

Adopt A Vegetarian Diet

Only a vegetarian diet is *sattvik*. Foods directly from the Mother Earth are modes of goodness. They increase the duration of life, purify one's existence and give strength, health, happiness and satisfaction. Such foods are juicy fruits, fatty, pleasing to heart, says Lord Krishna in the Bhagwad Gita-17.8

Keep Your Surroundings and Your Body Clean

Clean your house daily, wear clean clothes, and bathe at least once a day.

Indulge in Meaningful, Soulful Reads. Associate With People Having High *Sattvik* Energies:

When you will energize yourself with the higher vibrational energies, you will notice that the lower-frequency and the toxic people are suddenly disappearing from your life and the space is being created for high energetic vibrational people. The beautiful part of this is that you no longer miss the people who have left your life for good!

(Inspired by www.thesacredconnect.com)

Reasons For Fertility Issues In The Context of Three *Gunas*

There are couples who have no abnormal findings in their medical reports and have all-clear fertility status, yet fail to have kids. Why?

There are four basic reasons :

- The couple may be eligible for nurturing even a highly evolved being in their lives as their child, but their *tamsik, rajsik, sattvik* traits create hormonal imbalance, conceiving a baby, then, remains a big challenge . When the couples wish to turn their karmic relationship into a spiritual one, without any interference, they need to get out of the karmic loop by identifying their belief patterns, conditionings, and mindsets that are preventing them to evolve to an energetically blissful relationship. (This involves unconditional love, understanding and support. They need to rise above the need to have kids to evolve to a soulful relationship, feelings and bondage between them.

- For, when they have a karma with another soul, having give-and-take account, they may have to raise an adopted baby. Here, another couple or a single mother has to give birth to the child, but a different couple raises this baby. When this baby manifests in their lives, the resistance, sabotage is cleared, a soul-level forgiveness is granted and the couple may finally become eligible to have their own biological child.

- Female pathologies like ovarian cysts and benign tumours, blocked tubes, uterine structural abnormalities, such as fibroids, endometriosis, etc, happen at the base level for self-forgiveness, forgiveness for others and most important of all, acceptance of all, 'that is'. We shall discuss this in detail later in this book.

All the acquired major pathologies of the uterus-tubes-ovarian structures represent RESISTANCE in some form or the other-- resistance arising mainly due to lower vibrations of guilt, shame, fear, anger and victim consciousness.

You need to stop and ponder, which vibrations are you holding for long and creating resistance in the flow? When the dwelling on these lower vibrations goes for too long, it starts manifesting in the human body and the reproductive system, which turns dysfunctional, leading to a hindered conception.

THE STORY OF RUCHI SHAH NEW YORK, U.S.A.

Earlier this year, at 10:30pm, I was putting my busy day to rest and going through CWG part III when I received a call from my friend Mana in Mumbai (A highly evolved soul, hypnohealer, an Earth angel and the author of the book, Soul Song and 11:11)

It was a surprise call that reflected concern and urgency.

Her former client, Ruchi Shah, a clairvoyant and pregnant, had called from New York. She had been talking for a long time with the soul which wanted to come in, even before the pregnancy. She suddenly felt a break in the contact and knew intuitively that something was wrong.

I sensed another, lower vibrational soul, wanted to come, forcing its way in, due to earlier life family attachments. She saw the new soul pushing aside the one which had originally planned to come in. Ruchi was disturbed and anxious. What should she do? She wanted the original soul to come. They already had formed a bond.

Mana felt that I needed to be involved. I connected with Ruchi and with the consciousness of the unborn, we (Mana, Ruchi and I) saw or felt the same story—a soul was forcing it's way in, trying to convince the other soul to move on and take birth elsewhere, for its own growth. It was not serving anyone with its attachment to the family. For the highest good and growth of all and for the Earth, it needed to understand and seek it's evolution into unity elsewhere.

Ruchi is meant to bring in a new soul to Earth. She has been preparing her mind, body and soul to receive it. She had raised her vibrations through several modalities and with an effort in forgiveness and by creating joy and love.

The "bully soul" (lower vibrational one) had gate-crashed as it had found a leak in the energy vibrational level of this woman. It becomes very important and of immense value, therefore, to maintain and raise the energetic vibrations, so as to let the high soul to come in. Our ancient wisdom, drawn from the Vedas and other scriptures, describes in detail the "*pravarti*" or the "tendencies" of a soul (energy). Raising the *sattva guna tatva* is an easy way to purify the energetic system. As Ruchi consciously raised her *sattva* guna, not only did she retain the original soul as her forthcoming baby, but also sent unconditional love to the 'gate-crasher' soul , sending it to light and an incarnation most suitable for its evolution.

CHALLENGING FERTILITY

Why have we attracted it?

The assisted reproductive techniques, like IUI, IVF, ICSI, etc, have come in handy and gained much popularity. As a result, many childless couples are blessed parents now. The success rate, though, still is a mere 33%. A few IVF centers, however, claim to have it up to 40% or even more. These procedures generally include the spilling over of sperm near a well-developed ovum. ICSI, the procedure of injecting the sperm of highest quality inside the developed ovum is so direct and handy, but still the success rate is low!

Why?

Because, it is not just the body, the physical sperm and egg! It is the entire consciousness, the energetic system, of the egg and sperm which are at play. There is an existing electromagnetic field of the egg and the sperm, if the energies are not compatible, they become cancelling!

THE ENERGIES OF YOU TWO

The energy system of the female and that of the male, together, become the dominant energy systems of the gametes, the male and female reproductive cells (egg and sperm). On the superficial level, one may project oneself to be positive with happiness, belief and trust, but if subconscious mind remains in doubt, it is in the realm of highest probability, that one shall continue to have a doubtful outcome.

There can be several reasons: childhood episodes, or different intense stories which you have held for long as deeper vibrations inside your subconscious as you keep playing victim to these.

The most powerful addiction the humanity is used to, is the addiction to pain. This too is one choice which one may make repeatedly, i.e, choice to choose the pain.

In my experience through different workshops and regular fertility classes, the energetic cords and addictive patterns are found rooted deep in childhood memories and many a times in those nine months. Quite too often, when the would-be mothers go into their own intra-uterine periods, they find the cues, dissolve the knots and come back freed up.

It is high time you realize that your BODY is just the shape, size, colour, appearance, height of what you are, at the energetic, emotional, mental levels. It is the manifesting ground of the vibrations that you are, that you show up on the physical level as a reflection of who you are at the mental, emotional and spiritual levels.

Fibroid

(Due to) Guilt, **of not being enough.**

It is the guilt of previous miscarriages, abortions, energies of previous unsuccessful pregnancies still sitting in the womb, any womanly incompletions, guilt of creating unhappiness from childhood, discomfort to the parents, family members, guilt from any other past life episodes, etc, that may hound (Refer to the book, **Many Lives, Many Masters**, by Dr Brain Weiss, a renowned psychiatrist, where he proves the soul reincarnations.) This requires replacing the guilt with *FORGIVENESS*. One needs to forgive SELF before forgiving anyone else.

Adenomyosis

What, if infiltration and leakage of the life force happens in the direction not required, or not aligned with your life, and you are moving in the opposite direction? Have you ever made a self-sabotaging promise, or taken a vow in the past? These are the very strong energies of negation that generally obstruct the flow of life and the direction is often lost.

You need to go into your own self-journey and see if you are going against your own flow. If not, then, what is causing you so much pain? And why are you resisting it so much?

There is need for complete acceptance of the self and everyone else (especially your husband/partner). "As is" is the key. Letting go of the anger with full acceptance changes the flow to the desired, correct direction.

"Letting in", and completely accepting motherhood, will sail you through, even if you are not pregnant yet.

Blocked/Absent tubes
Karmic/ resistance, resistance at the soul level

It is generally one or more of the following:

1. Fear (of the outcome)
2. Doubt (if it is going to work at all)
3. Anger (self-anger and low self-esteem of not been able to bear a child)
4. Victim consciousness (Blame that "my destiny holds this", or "it's my husband's fault", or some other reason)

These vibrations and energies hardly ever will work in your favour. Hence, the negative results!

Various Ovarian Cysts Or Tumours

If the ovaries are present and they are present with follicles within them, you are a strong candidate as are the billion others on the planet, to at least produce a healthy, fertilizable egg.

If your body and its systems are not helping your ovaries to mature, there surely is a blockage. Let me explain this : imagine there is a bathroom and the tank overhead is filled with water (your hypothalamus gland, *crown chakra*, from where all supply and the super regulation of hormones take place) and the tank is connected through pipes to supply water (for hormonal balance and release of the egg) to various taps and the shower. When the outflow from the tap is on, i.e, the tubes are patent, the shower is ready to let the water sprinkle out, it will and you will enjoy a great bath under the shower outlet. Would it happen that there is a great supply from the tank, but the shower is still not spilling water? There has to be some blockage, somewhere in the systems of pipes/ or at the level of the shower outlet itself, if the water flow is missing.

The pores may be blocked because of the continued non-supply of water and ultimate clogging, but is this the core reason for the water supply to be absent? No.

Is it the blocked pores which are the reason for non-supply? No.

That, in fact, is the RESULT of long-standing no supply of water.

There is certainly a block at some other level. What will happen if we keep on cleansing the pores of the outlet and not deal with the real blockage? The pores will block again due to the persisting no supply!

Similarly, the cysts or tumours which may be simple haemorrhagic or endometriotic cysts of various sizes, shapes and complexities stand as the blocked pores at the shower outlet! They are the RESULT of the blockages elsewhere.

Only dealing with the correction of these cysts and tumours generally at the local level does not resolve the problems and often they come back (just like the blockage of pores of the shower outlet comes back).

These ovarian cysts and tumours are a result of sabotages and hence the blockages are elsewhere! They certainly are not the *root* of the problem. To reach the root we need to dig up deeper and find out the real points of creation of these blockages.

Clearing these blockages will result in the opening of the blockages. The patency will be achieved and the outflow will be excellent without any recurrence of any ovarian obstacles.

This sounds easy, and it is easy. The easiness depends upon the level of your conviction, faith, belief and the *"will"* to resolve. The doubts and skepticism will keep your pores blocked, as they have been doing for a long time now.

The power to resolve and dissolve anything and everything unserving lies within you. It is high time you acknowledge, embrace and execute it.

Therefore, recall the sound of **'AAEE'** and remind yourself what it stands for :

A - Acknowledge
A - Accept
E - Embrace
E – Execute

Whenever the sound of "AAEE" comes out of your mouth, you need to have firm belief in what these four letters stand for and, surrender, with full faith and hope, what we call *astha* and *asha* in Hindi translation. It is high time for you to let go of the control and surrender to the power of cosmic energies and let the magic play and miracles happen.

WHEN MAGIC PLAYS, THE MIRACLES HAPPEN!

Here, I can't emphasize enough when I say this. Only working on the physical, dense aspects usually doesn't leave us with much good! Another important factor which comes into play is the super cancellation or super imposition of energies.

How can you alter the electromagnetic field of the two gamete cells, so that the zygote and then the embryo and hence the baby which is formed is a **prodigy**?

Let us understand this with an anology, that of a queen bee. Several labour bees (sperms) are ready to impregnate the queen bee, but only the one with the correct, corresponding electromagnetic field will approach her(egg) and the one with perfect (lock and key) electromagnetic effect will be able to impregnate. The ratio generally is of 1: 80 million, i.e, 60 to 80 million sperms are required to fertilize a single ovum with a single most aligned, suitable sperm(in cases of natural conception to occur)

Still no conception?

The perfect life code will happen when the energetic superimposition has taken place. This may take up to one year for a couple to conceive. Couples with the right frequencies and intentions are able to produce results very quickly.

THE THEORY OF PERFECT CONCEPTION

If we do an aura photography of a sperm and egg, we see how they are similar and in what way they differ. The similar ones often have a high potential of conception and the dissimilar ones do not fertilize.

What is an electromagnetic field?

It is described as a physical force produced by an electrically charged object. Whenever electricity is passed through a metallic object, it forms an electromagnetic field around it. Similarly, the human electric impulse in the brain and throughout the nervous system, through your body, creates an electromagnetic field. Billions of nerve impulses, negative and positive discharges in form of negative and positive emotions, add to this electromagnetic field.

The electromagnetic field, i.e, aura of the gametes need to be accepting to each other for the penetration (impregnation) to happen. These auras/electromagnetic fields have to be complementing to each other.

They are a reflection of your body's cumulative aura. One of the major causes and concerns of infertility are or could be the opposing/contradicting electromagnetic fields of the human body and hence the human gametes.

But the good news is that this aura or the electromagnetic field is ever-changing and could be influenced. It is a perfect and complete reflection of your inner world. The aura or the electromagnetic field is a reflection of your CORE, which consists of :

1. Emotions - Primarily
2. Beliefs
3. Attitudes
4. Hopefulness
5. Willingness

Causes of 'no conception', as discussed before, hence, may be :

1. Mechanical hindrances.
2. Physical challenges, diseases of the reproductive systems, the sexuality issues, dysfunctions and hormonal imbalances , in the highest possibility, are the result of the un-matching, un-lockable CORE.

For you to shift your core, you have to be willing to undergo changes in your emotions, hopefulness, beliefs and attitudes. By bringing about the desired changes, not only does your body's electromagnetic field change, but also that of the gametes.

The similar changes in the core lead to a shift in the electromagnetic fields (aura) of the couple, thereby influencing the electromagnetic fields of the gametes positively, further raising the possibility of acceptance of the two cells. Both male and female cells now have a harmony of changes and the conception may happen.

THE ENERGY TRANSFORMATION, POST CONCEPTION

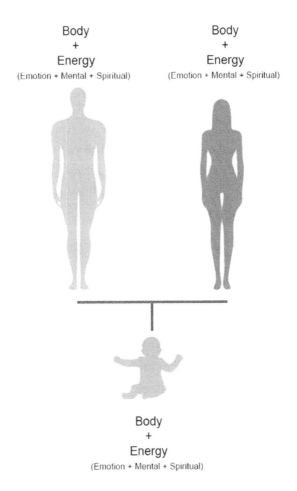

Body
+
Energy
(Emotion + Mental + Spiritual)

Body
+
Energy
(Emotion + Mental + Spiritual)

Body
+
Energy
(Emotion + Mental + Spiritual)

The concept that I am to share now is very much inherent to our consciousness. It is not only integral to our knowledge that we use in our day-to-day lives, but sadly, is not part of our lives as it is not much in awareness.

You know this and have learnt well at school.

Energies cannot be created, nor can they be destroyed;
they can just be transformed from one form to another.
Multi-cellular, trillions of cells and the cosmic truth

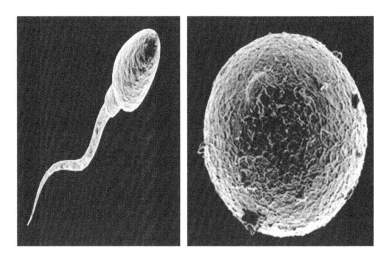

Single cell + Single cell

We have learnt about mitosis and meiosis at school, the procedures of cell division and multiplication by cell replication and genetic transformation of information, carried inside the DNA.

But what about the energetic part of it, especially when the cells are coming together?

The energy contained by a single sperm has kinetic energy, potential energy and a lot more. There is some momentum with which it enters the ovum, trying impregnating it. The ovum is at inertia, having a lot of potential energy.

Kinetic Energy + Potential Enery Momentum(To Hit the ovum with Mass X) + Potential Energy(egg)

Hence, a zygote is formed which has $K.E_1 + P.E_1 + P.E_2$

Here, p1 and k1 are the kinetic energies of the sperm and PE2 is the potential energy of the ovum.

But are these energies of the two cells enough to crop 50 trillion cells to the forthcoming human body? The answer is 'yes'. In fact, it is a lot more!

The energy inputs are received from the mother's body through food, water, air and space(impacts from external environment) and love, faith, surrender, courage, bliss, doubt, guilt, anger, pride, fear, etc., (impacts from internal environment) all of these comprise the unique electromagnetic field or the aura of sperm and egg.

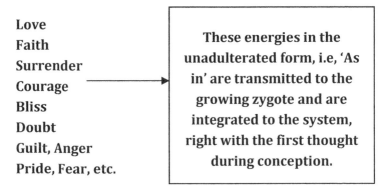

Love
Faith
Surrender
Courage
Bliss
Doubt
Guilt, Anger
Pride, Fear, etc.

These energies in the unadulterated form, i.e, 'As in' are transmitted to the growing zygote and are integrated to the system, right with the first thought during conception.

Evidently, you will give your best to your incoming unborn, so you need to acquire and release a lot, becoming the best version of yourself!

This phase of blueprint shall continue throughout the period while your baby is inside you and by the time the baby is delivered, and later until it grows up to 8-9 years of life. The energies from mother, father, grandparents, other family members, neighbourhood members, and the society, cumulatively transmit energy and the active subconscious mind programming takes place continuously.

So the "being" that is created is not just the physical cells taking the shape of head, eyes, face, heart, chest, abdomen, feet and hands. It is constantly receiving bundles of different frequencies of energies, including the emotional ones, much of which are transmuted every millisecond. These energies contribute to the basic conditionings and nature of the upcoming human being, hence so much of variety. The permutation and combination of several emotional energies actually cumulate to the unique formula of this particular being, i.e, your fetus , your unborn baby.

So, now imagine the superpower, the power house that the mother is! **The mother has the power to create a God, a Demon, a Human, or an Animal !**

This, of course, depends upon the mental, emotional and situational conditioning of the mother.

With the perfect awareness each and every aspiring mother/already a mother has this boundless potential to recondition herself NOW and change the configuration of energetic reactions which her body is calibrating and minutely monitor the 'SELF' transmission.

The Mother Is the "Superpower" On The Planet Earth.

THE ENERGY AND THE LIFE

The Thought leads to the creation.

The very thought of the sacred act, the very basic instinct to life and survival is the transmission and conversion of energies. Here, the energy is represented by a wave.

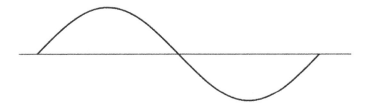

This wave has an amplitude.

The energies show compliance, correspondence and flow , when in the same direction. The superimposition of the energies creates a total increase in the energetic surge. This surge and exponential increase in the energy wave amplitude due to superimposition of like energies often lead to a favourable conception. With this high surge, all positive, enhanced energy is transformed to the upcoming zygote.

The future foetus and hence the future infant rises and encapsulates the high energy encryption. High energy here does not mean physical high energy, but the energies of positivity, productivity, such as trust, love, faith and surrender, full of ecstatic encrypted code. The energy code opens up as the foetus is born and a proper programme, i.e, a message is offered to the just born fetus, especially during the first six hours of the birth. This code is fully loaded. And hence, *the blueprint to the future is created.*

The energy bundle becomes the foundation of life and the subconscious programme becomes the structure in the first couple of years of your infant's life.

PRODUCTIVE

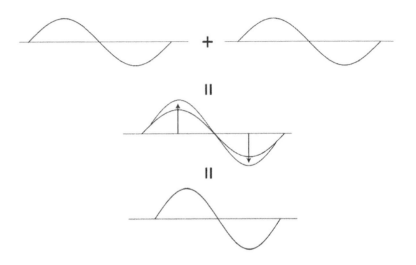

On the other hand,

If the act performed between two people is with opposite energies, embodying low and high energy levels, what happens is this:

UNPRODUCTIVE

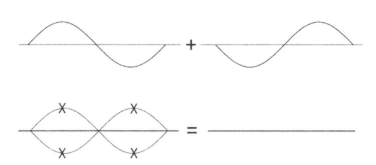

It depends upon the energy level at that moment. If the energy is not compatible for a conception, cancellation at the amplitude happens (the peak point of the energetic wave), the amplitudes do not superimpose, but cancel each other. The foundation is almost a straight line, i.e., the energy code is lifeless.

Such conceptions generally do not happen. Even if the conception does happen, it mostly results in the formation of abnormal fetuses (improper structure erection because of a very weak or no foundation).

Such babies, if at all they come, will be prone to having

- Weak personalities
- Diseases
- Lack of self-confidence
- Low value system
- Low love quotient
- Low faith levels

Let us note that,

- When two people are planning to have a baby consciously, or even those who have landed into an accidental conception, the energetic sync of these two people is a must, very vital for the future child blueprinting. I am frequently asked a very valid question on this: So, why do conceptions happen out of rape? Answer is the same, because of the energetic sync, energies of fear, deep anger and rage are common in both gametes.
- Even if the energies are appropriate, but the thought process at that given moment is not in sync, the resulting energetic bundle will not be so appropriate so as to form a very strong foundation. A pre-conceptual planning is as vital a programme as a mother's need to feed herself for the growth of the baby.

RESOLVING KARMA

Once the patterns are identified after the awareness is created, it is time to identify the karmic relationship, time to resolve the karma between two people involved. If the karma is released both ways, your relationship moves to another grid or level of experiences, which is in the highest of you both and with your free will, if you choose to. If the release is from one side, and the other person still chooses to experience the same karma, he or she will manifest someone else to have similar experiences, until he or she decides to integrate the lesson and move forward!

Hence, it is most advisable to strengthen that level, seal the energy leak there, overcome and muster that emotion and move upwards with a pure, connected and loving experience with the same human being. If both are not willing, they attract someone else who is ready and programmed to be at that energetic level, and in sync with your life purpose.

Even if one is primarily vibrating at a higher consciousness like the level of love and above, an unresolved karma, or a low frequency minor leak (echo) can lead to an emotional fluctuation and lowering of vibration. This can trigger the emotional response, unless the karma is resolved (or/ and an awareness is Created → Identified → Replaced → Upgraded).

Through accessing body consciousness (ABC), by Sidra Jafri, at the energetic level and at the level of consciousness, the relationship with people around us dramatically improves or those people (our triggers, who help us realize our emotional leaks and echoes) leave us and our environment or we become neutral towards them, as their karma has been fulfilled.

There is always another level to be at, always another layer to be peeled off. One must understand that though there is no urgency to fulfill or do anything, it all is about being present. It is about being fully aware to flow with the flow completely and totally. All that "is" shall manifest, and when it does, we just have to let it be, by completely surrendering to faith and the flow. When the energetic manifestations happen with the highest order of faith --- MAGIC AND MIRACLES show up! Remember, beyond 8% of our conscious mind, in the deeper layers of 92% subconscious, lie the Faith, Magic and Miracle !

THE LIGHT AS A CHANNEL OF TRANSFORMATION

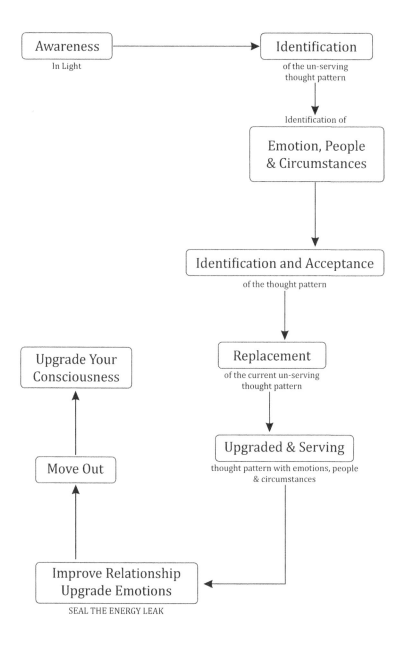

FAITH

Key to unlock the subconsciousness to unleash the
miracles to happen and magic to unfold

Why Motherhood/ Parenthood?

"When you've tried lifting the mountains, done with doing all that
you could and still there where you were, more tortured, more
confused, more skeptical, more anxious, disappointed and above all
with more of remorse and despair, almost as if the hope is lost, give
me (divine) a chance and just leave things to me and sit back all
relaxed (if you can) – just Non-intervening."

Feel that the magic is all around.

After 19+ years of medical practice, especially while dealing with
mothers and would-be mothers, one thing I am fully convinced of--
that there are patterns on this journey, the patterns of learning,
unlearning, breaking and embracing. These are unique patterns
and realities.

Motherhood happens at a divine time, when we are ready to let go
of something that is un-serving and let in something more serving.

Each pregnancy gets with it a strong set of emotions, feelings,
hopes and anxieties. These nine months are a crucial period to
change the grid.

All that is un-serving is reflected, especially in the initial three
months, and you mostly push out your old un-serving belief
patterns, karmic conditionings and past-life memories, as they
surface layer by layer.

There is a medical condition, called hyperemesis gravidarium, i.e, excessive vomiting during pregnancy. This widely studied condition has full medical back-up, pathophysiological explanation and medical treatment. We as doctors find ourselves often saying, 'This will happen for first 3 months mostly, then it will pass off and settle down. Medicines will, of course, help you recover, but when you miss a single dose, it all comes back. In severe cases, no medicine helps! Hospitalization, injectables and IV fluids become the only remedy."

This time is perfect to reflect upon the emotions, feelings, and patterns which have come up during this energetic intervention, your baby inside you is a brand new energetic system your body is trying to adjust with!. Your newly acquired energy seems to be a catalyst, a mirror to look into ourselves at a deeper level, and this is the time to transform.

Your new embryo inside you certainly is a medium to a plethora of spiritual and energetic enhancements if, of course, you are willing to accept and flow with it. Your resistance will only result in the deepening of suffering, excessive symptomatology, fear, anxiety about the outcome and one may land up struggling sometimes in hospital or even end up losing the babies.

If we talk about missed abortions, blighted ovum, spontaneous abortions or even recurrent pregnancy loss, RPL when the patterns simply re-occur during each pregnancy, if not dealt with and not healed, it all comes back in the same pregnancy loss pattern time and again. Hence, we find ourselves caught in the vicious cycle of this loop.

We shall speak about the metaphysical or energetic part of the challenges of the first trimester in detail later on in the next part of this book.

THE STORY OF MEERJAHAN

Haridwar, Uttarakhand
A chronicle unbelievable

Married for 6 years in her late twenties, face withered with early wrinkles and pain, hurt and guilt written all over the woman, called Meerjahan, her husband was a contrast, standing high, a lively figure of confidence and hope.

YEAR: 2012

They had first came to me with the woman's condition, called severe endometriosis complaining of difficult, painful cycles, heavy flow during cycles and inability to conceive, her internal pelvic body structures were adherent to each other. She had been on medication, almost ever since she had married.

Her last hope was a surgical removal of adhesions to free up her structures as much as possible. Good, that she was not so educated and did not even try to understand the complicated medical terminologies and pathophysiologies. We took her for surgery. Her entire pelvis, tubes, ovaries and uterus were badly stuck to each other. Doing any surgical intervention posed a hazard of an uncontrolled bleeding, so we did what was ideal in this condition: closed her abdomen back. She was beyond any surgical repair.

This was four years ago. Now, her only hope was IVF or surrogacy, which, they simply could not afford, so they opted for another divine option, called *adoption*. They adopted a baby girl. With this, she adopted a LIFE for her!

YEAR: 2015

Meerjahan, once again entered my chamber, holding a three-year-old girl. She was very happy, beautiful and a charming child. I had not seen Meerjahan so happy ever before. Her face glowed with candour, she seemed so calmed and relaxed, not leaving her daughter's hand, holding her apparently with deep love, compassion and contentment

Logic was doing rounds in my brain, remembering her history and her case study. A logical conclusion could be that her problems had worsened in these three years of relentless medication and that she must be in the deepest possible pain ever? But my intuitive side did discover something better: I was smelling a miracle! And she soon stated, exactly what I was brooding over : "Madam, I am in the 3rd month of my pregnancy."

WHAT?

"Really?" My mind went jostling. "But your tubes were stuck and pelvis was in a bad shape, how could you....?"

"HOW?"

This has, however, never been in our understanding and in our hands. So we better park all that aside.

But the truth is that in spite of every obstacle she faced, Meerjahan was *pregnant*. After her daughter came into her life, all her skepticism, anxieties, disappointments and fear got washed away as she observed the most powerful law of Nature :

The law of Gratitude

She thanked Almighty day and night for the blessings. The motherhood had got to her that she was eternally happy, joyful and peaceful with the gift or gifts and that her life was now enough and fulfilled.

This feeling of being contented and having enough had qualified her to receive much more than she had ever expected.

WHY ME OF ALL THE PEOPLE ON THIS PLANET?

Prayer for the evolved soul: "I invite a rainbow soul or a highly evolved soul in my life as our child, with a healthy beautifully formed body, high intelligence, high level of awareness and consciousness. I willingly allow this soul to follow its highest path, willingly support and understand the higher purpose of this birth, and stay committed to help bloom and blossom midway. And so it is."

The very topic of this chapter reflects how I have been doubtful and skeptical. "How?" has been my favourite question ever since. Many of you may identify with this, and many may feel the same at this moment. "How can a skeptical person write a chapter on this topic ?" And..."Why on earth am I reading it?"

Why me, of all the people who have embarked upon this journey in this manner and have chosen to undergo these particular sets of experiences?

This sprouts out of the inherent desire of our *core*--ourselves at heart, to know, identify, adapt, and assimilate. There is no one way on the journey of faith, if at all we decide to embark on it. Of course, we are tested, but who cares if we are in complete faith and surrender?

Faith and doubt, are sharply contrasting, aren't they? We need faith to overcome our doubts and completely surrender. Our logical minds cannot and are not in a position to comprehend the act of faith and surrender. It is beyond logic, as are miracles and magic!

Now, let's dive into daytime, imagination, dreaming stuff. We are super active at imagining things and visit places where we have never gone or even know if they exist at all. Let us do it !

Imagine this entire universe, several galaxies, our own galaxy with infinite stars and planets and their solar systems, our solar system, then this beautiful planet of ours and this huge world population of 7.5 billion people. Then, imagine you and your partner and then that one soul that you have attracted in your life as your baby or your developing foetus inside you...

Is it a mere coincidence?

This energetic combination of you people--you, your partner and your baby, is the "most" on this planet at any given moment of time.

These sacred groups, unique combinations, permutations and sets of energies choose to come together. There could be no other way. It was meant to be.

why?

Here, we may have a logical explanation. Are you ready? If yes, then read this:

We, as human beings are not just *bodies*. Just as current passes through an iron piece, it becomes a magnet, similarly, when the life force or the energy (current) passes through your body (iron piece), you become magnetic.

There are different frequencies or vibrations at which one vibrates (as explained before). The amount of life force, the pace at which it is passing through you, the very condition of your body (how much disease-free, healthy are you how much wear-and-tear has already been done) defines your own magnetic properties.

We witness it everywhere around us, all the time. There are people of very ordinary looks who always shine, come may what, and become the centre of mass attention. And there are people who, no matter how physically attractive they are, sit timid and withdrawn, not making their presence felt in crowds. This is all about the level of magnetism that your "*beingness*" oozes out of you. The good news is this is changeable, achievable and attainable!

Coming back to the former, depending upon our energetic emission at that given moment, we attract another energetic emission in our lives, the baby we attract is directly dependent upon our own energetic state. It is entirely in our hands to choose what we want to experience through our kids as we manifest or attract them energetically in our lives.

There are highly evolved souls who are waiting and willing for the right energetic and physical combinations as human beings at the right magnetic amplitude, so that they can enter the space and find appropriate environment to be in, and let their bodies develop inside.

Lower vibrations like guilt, shame, anger, fear, apathy, suspicion, doubt, at the time of conception will attract souls which resonate with these vibrations. If you are suffering with hypertension, diabetes, heart problem, infectious diseases, like tuberculosis, etc, hormonal disturbances at the time of conception, definitely low energy souls will be attracted in your life--which most of the times is the case. It qualifies you to have an insecure, fearful, anxious, angry and a doubtful soul as your child.

This came out as a huge revelation to me. What is the need for the excitement when the kid is born ? Why do you look forward to astrological prediction? You know what you have *created and crafted* after all, from moment to moment to moment and organ to organ. You know beforehand what you have created and how that is going to unfold in future! And I happens exactly this way.

Your wealth, position in the society, social, political power and fame, do not matter at all. That explains exactly why we see the rise of a commoner's child and failure of a very successful and famous person's child.

We cannot buy bodies (we can certainly pay for their repair) and we certainly cannot buy the energies, we can only attract these energies. There are life forces, directly proportional to the personality we reflect in our real lives at theat particular point of time.

And this concept applies to your husband or wife too. The combination of the energetic, physical existence of you both is going to determine the physical and energetic composition of your baby.

It entirely depends on you and who you allow to affect yourself? How much power do you retain with you and how much do you give away?

You only need to pause from this never-ending race of life that we are running and ask the following questions to yourself:

You, on a scale of 0-10, write down the first number that comes to your mind.

	Score
• How happy am I in my current situation of life?	
• Where am I physically health wise?	
• Where am I emotionally, how balanced am I?	
• How much do I blame others, environment or even God?	
• How much do I justify my acts to others?	
• How much complaining am I about self, family, environment, government, system, pollution and God?	
• How healthy are my relationships?	
• How strong am I mentally?	
• How strongly have I held my past to myself?	
• How anxious am I for the future?	
• How much am I able to live in the present moment with full awareness?	
• How much faith have I in the infinite intelligence of God or the Universe?	
• How much am I surrendered with peace and calmness?	
• How much am I able to be fully present, be fully aware in a given moment of time?	
• How relaxed am I as to everything being absolutely fine in my universe?	
• How easily am I able to give and receive?	

You have to give a number that first comes to your mind : 0 means absolutely nothing, 10 means complete compliance. Any area which is less than 6 or equal to 6, needs attention and can be improved upon.

"All that we seek, seeks us"

In a most simplified manner, all that is needed for a child , at the subtle energetic level, is a womb and an appropriate environment, around that womb, for that energy to sustain, bloom and evolve inside you.

Now, let us peruse this example:

How many of you love green plants and are indulgent about growing indoor plants?

These beautiful flowering plants, with good fragrances, need good soil, nurturing and a daily dose of sunlight for the colours to come up bright and beautiful!

What will happen, with you having cleaned the soil of all weeds, adding the needed fertilizers, doing all very well after planting, but giving very little water and almost no sun exposure? Even if the soil is great and the plant is of high quality, the full bloom will not happen and, as a result, the plant may even die down in the process of growing up.

Similarly, even after cleansing your bodies at the physical, emotional, mental, spiritual levels, if the consistency is not maintained in thoughts and actions, the imbalance will occur. The cleansing will attract a beautiful, rich soul in your lives, but if you drop your awareness and consciousness and disturb the internal environment, the soul, troubled by the inhospitable, contradicting environment, to be in , may resolve to leave your body mid-way, resulting in an intra-uterine death. This may happen through sudden leakage through the water bag, bleeding or a sudden loss of fetal movement. These are the signs and symptoms of a disturbed, imbalanced, internal environment which may not be acceptable to the incoming high order soul that, in turn, may contemplate leaving .

If a child is conceived out of compulsive sex, anger, frustration, guilt, shame or criminal assault, it is generally observed that these pregnancies are strong in nature. Even if the mother tries hard to abort through different home remedies or medicines, abortions become difficult. This is because the mother has attracted a very low frequency soul to her system, which needs lower vibrations or emotions, such as shame, guilt, apathy, despair and anger to survive. These pregnancies go well until term and are delivered healthily. On a further research, it has come to light that these children are generally a challenge to foster, not honest, frustrated, angry and lack compassion. These children generally give a tough time to their parents.

So, with your emotions, feelings and thoughts during your ongoing pregnancy, you can easily know who you have attracted as your baby and what could be his or her future like!

THE TIME UNTIL YOU CONCEIVE

You certainly aren't aware of exactly how and when is it most appropriate and fruitful to have that baby or energy as yours. Maybe, it will happen whenever it is meant to be and you would simply let it be, maybe, you will have challenges in conceiving as your friend or a friend's friend is facing?.

Maybe?

Here you may put yourselves into the bracket of being a victim as you feel powerless or at the receiving end. Why?

- Do you feel that you are the creator?
                    OR
- Do you feel that you are functioning under the influence of the choices made by others for you?
- Let me come back to what I have said earlier :
- You have a choice to exactly attract the new soul/ baby in your life.
- You exactly are in control of "the choice" of who (here "who" refers to the energy of your kid, it does not refer to the sex of the baby) you are going to have as your baby.
- And that you are powerful enough to create and co-create the exact environment required for the subtle soul to be in, attracted as your baby.

We've all grown witnessing the effect and impact of our external environment which a person is in, at any given moment of time and at any place on the planet. *This is the universal law of existence.*

Your environment is always more powerful than you, says T Harv Eker.

Our internal environment is a direct reflection of our external environment and the latter is a direct mirror- image of our internal environment, i.e,

Internal environment ∝ External environment

Both these worlds are the mirror-images of each other. Not to mention that both are an illusion and perception of one's mind. Nevertheless, we perceive them as real.

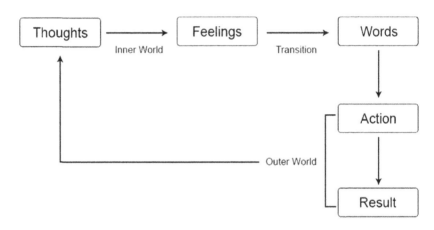

Let me explain this,

We all know that we, at the basic level, are all energy and a cumulative energy source. Our entire body is made up of organ systems

- Organ Tissues Cells Molecule Atom Sub atomic particles

Electron Proton Neutron

We, at the core level are bundles of energy just vibrating and anything that is energy, when passed through the current (life force/ will) produces an electromagnetic field. You may also qualify to have that "Halo" that the Zen-masters and the Gods have, it is just that we need to be a little more enlightened, i.e, fill ourselves with light!

When the life force (the cosmic life energy or *"Prana"*) enters the energy field of your 'awake' physical body, which itself is a cluster of vibrating sub-atomic particles at the quantum level and produces light, it is then you start becoming full of it, i.e., begin the journey to enlightenment. This journey is full of courage and unconditional love.

To understand this, let's reflect on this box

Spiritual	**Mental**
Emotional	**As a body Physical Manifestation**

Whatever is cooking up in these other 3 bodies, shows up in the physical body.

It is like organizing a perfect dinner. You first go to grocery, buy vegetables, wash them and finally cut and cook them. The cooking will not happen unless there is a catalyst of heat even if all ingredients, including water and spices, are put together in the required proportion. Similarly, our ingredients are mental thoughts, emotional feelings, heat--the catalyst--is the spiritual energy, i.e, very basic energy of one's existence. When all these align in a particular combination, the final dinner table, your physical body is laid out.

This dinner is not random as the preparation, ingredients, recipes, heat and labour have all been put into it. Similarly, we do not exist randomly, our physical body, health, illnesses , pain, aches, beauty, condition of each and every internal organ, nerve, muscle, fiber, is a direct consequence of all our states put together.

> Spiritual
> Emotional   ⟶   State= Physical State
> Mental

What we as humans focus on is the very physical body with ailments and diseases. While our bodies only mirror and reflect what actually exists beneath and within.

What happens when you polish and paint a wooden door which is bugged with termite? No matter how beautifully, expensively and diligently you have polished or painted, the termite will still feast on the wood. Similarly, we keep visiting doctors for ailments for various chronic diseases like, diabetes, hypothyroidism hypertension (high B.P.), heart ailments, obesity, recurring heal aches, backaches, spinal problems, kidney diseases, stomach ailments, asthma, allergies, various cysts, female genital problems, infertility of varying origins, recurring UTI...the list is endless..

We keep polishing and painting our termite-ridden bodies time and again, changing the colours and qualities of paints and polishes from time-to-time, but for how long does it last?

How often do you get cured? Or better still, do you ever get cured? How many times do the symptoms go, just to come back soon?

How much is the chance that you will be off your medicines forever?

We can't deny and applaud enough, the breakthrough researches that our scientists have carried out, and we as doctors, offer quick remedies, fixing methods for our physical bodies, relieving us of our pains. But, where are the cures? How often does a patient, of a chronic ailment, actually is declared healthy and is put off medication?

Any disease will first perceive the disturbance, both at the mental and emotional levels. This deep-seeded emotional charge creates the energy disturbance at the mental level and then cumulatively these disturbed energies from all these levels manifest at the physical body level.

Why do we open our eyes only when there is a final knock at the weak, superficially polished- painted termite-laden door?

Why not have a strong, termite resistant-door in the first place?

The answer obviously is 'ok.'

But, HOW?

There are several techniques through which we can now identify the default--spiritual, mental and emotional malfunctions-- correct them and have a cleaned shiny, disease-free body.

No wonder, the saints, sages and more disciplined people who live high up in the mountains, without much of medical assistance, can draw breath to a hundred years!

Impossible? Nah! Are they humans? Yes, very much .

But they are sages, living up somewhere...

So? Arn't they humans?

Arn't you one?

You MOST certainly don't need to become a sage or climb up mountains to find your light..

Then what and HOW ?

You will not find it anywhere externally, because you carry it inside of you !

Remember the deer and its musk ?..

Pause for a moment , close your eyes, take a few deep breaths in, and now ask yourself...

Show me my light

Be there. You may see something or you may not, but rest assured, you have just knocked at your inner door, so there will be a response.

Keep on asking yourself this, until you are answered. You shall have it only when you are ready to receive.

Now, coming back to the point of concern.

YOU, on way to becoming parents :

The 'like' energy people at the core attract, and unlike ones repel. One may show off as whatever one wishes to, at the superficial physical level, thanks to conscious thinking, which knows how to pretend and mask the true self. An angry person, who will charge up at the slightest trigger, at any point of time, may or may not have an angry life partner. This person will most likely be a silently angry soul, whose life's purpose will be to experience anger, through you.

So, it is entirely up to you, to attract whatever you wish to, but for that, you have to choose your energetic, mental, and emotional system.

Easy? You bet!

Let us also understand how you will perform this chosen act, and energetically raise your vibrations. There is a concept that needs to be explored and understood.

Let's talk about our mind. It can be, for our understanding, divided into the conscious and the subconscious. Our conscious mind is just 6-8%. It is the creative, understanding and the wise mind. Here, all the learning, unlearning, analysis and creation take place. This is a beautiful thing to be with. The things are changeable with thoughts, feelings and emotions. Our subconscious mind (s/c mind) is a "habituated mind". Once a habit is created, it will just be repeated, it has no logic, no good or bad sense, no wisdom, no affection, no emotion and no feeling. This is just like a tape recorder which will keep on playing the music that has been recorded on the tape, whether the audience likes it or not, whether or not an audience is there at all. It will just play and replay, of course, until we switch it off !

So, when you have a programme from past experiences or thoughts like "pregnancy is difficult, dangerous, unpredictable, labour pain is unbearable, there are several diseases of the pregnancy congenital anomaly", or the worst of all, if you have witnessed a death due to maternity, delivery, you have seen someone trying hard to conceive, but has mostly encountered disappointment and chronic infertility, your fears will firmly set in-- that these stories will be your future stories. Thus, habitual visualization (remember visualization with emotion form a strong subconscious belief or a subconscious programme) takes place and you tread on similar problems.

DIVINITY IN CONCEPTION, HOW?

What is it that you search in your life?

What are your unfulfilled desires, where in your life do you feel something is missing ?

The very act of conception is an act of spirituality. Do you have it at your discretion? Culminate this act and turn it into conception? Togetherness is your choice, but conception happens at the divine time. You unconsciously become a part of this spiritual process, not understanding much and generally come to know about the news of the pregnancy not until a few days have passed, that you have conceived, and sometimes even later!

You become channel and medium for divinity to express itself. The universe does not distinguish between rich and poor, lethargic and hard-working, healthy or sick, working or non-working, hateful or loving, cruel or compassionate, it just functions on certain set principles and universal laws.

The law of karma is what is being played here.

Karma has nothing to do with morality. It is simple cause and effect.

What you sow, so shall you reap !

We embark on an all the new dimension of our spiritual journey through conception, the most spiritual enhancing landmark of your lifetime. Seemingly insignificant, unimportant, almost random, but significantly a turning points of your life.

When you are ready to undergo yet another spiritual or karmic cycle, you unconsciously let the pregnancy happen to you. Our conscious mind, logical thinking is all put to rest.

For now, go back into your memory and try to remember your first reaction to the news of your pregnancy?

- Was it doubt?
- Was it fear?
- Was it insecurity?
- Was it, "Oh, too early?"
- Was it utter happiness?
- Or, the surge of love and gratitude?

These responses are the first step towards blueprinting your child for a lifetime. I take a look back to Feb '99, when I got the news of my first. At that time, my husband was pursuing his post-graduation degree and I was in my first year of residency in a government hospital in Delhi. We were living in a post graduade hostel accommodation.

My first reaction was, "What will happen?"

This reaction come from an energy to control everything in my environment (to which, many of you may resonate) and our inherent nature to doubt as we use our logical thinking too often and too much. It took a while for me to let the fact sink in and when it did, there were the next set of doubts, waiting to show up.

Just peruse your first reactions and you shall know exactly the note at which this life-transforming journey, called pregnancy, has begun.

THE POWER OF WORDS

We, as human beings, are structured and conditioned on ancient beliefs and patterns. We carry the past memories of grief, suppression, capping and limiting ourselves, with doubt, struggling mostly for survival in competition with one another. The very thought that goes in the "beingness" is competition for survival which gets carried forward to home with siblings, at school, family, cousins and at college. The combative thought travels further to relationships, between spouses and then we grandly pass it on to the next generation. What, if we take the initiative to stop and turn around this vicious cycle from, "There is a lot of competition", to "I am enough, I am unique, I am who I am?"

What, if the word competition gets replaced by the word cooperation?

What, if our day-to-day vocabulary consists of the following words frequently used by us?

FAITH	COMPASSION	HONESTY
TRUST	LOVE & PASSION	FAIRNESS
BLISS	POWER	JOY
GRACE	ABUNDANCE	MERCY
COOPEARTION	SUPPORT	COURAGE

- Just feel the power of these words now!

  Take a moment out for yourself. Close your eyes, get into the present moment, be aware of your surroundings. Take three breaths. And just repeat these words in relation to your pregnancy. How do these words make you feel?

_____

_____

_____

_____

_____

- Our connection with the outer world is through our words. What is the impact of these words on your thoughts?

_____

_____

_____

_____

_____

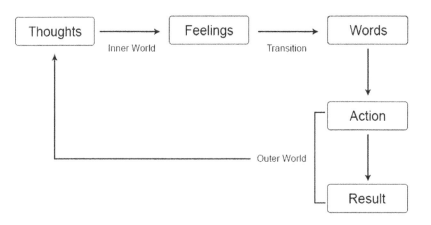

Now, choose negative words, such as, hatred, competition, jealousy, anger, frustration, fear, shame, grief, despair, curse, depression, rivalry, greed, pain, murder and so forth, and speak them up !

How do you feel now?

You will realize that by merely speaking out these words had an impact on you.

I, therefore, suggest the following:

Choose words of high energy, positive energy and integrate them at your basic core memory and feel your electromagnetic field-- aura oozing out the energy of these words.

With such vibrations in your magnetic aura, who are you going to invite as your baby?

Just think about it!

THE STORY OF JASPREET

Jaspreet, a 24-year-old woman, pursuing her nursing degree was into her first pregnancy. She was living with her husband in a faraway land to earn a living. She had a big joint family to adjust with, along with this ongoing pregnancy.

Jaspreet had to adjust with somewhat hostile environment at the in-laws' place. The men in the household lived with profoundly abusive language. Most utterances started with Hindi slangs and abusive words and ended with them. Women were noticeably docile, immensely frustrated and were hardly allowed to express!

Jaspreet wanted her baby to be full of virtues. She was particularly fearful of the slangs that the baby might catch up. She joined the classes and the workshop that we offer. We taught her the technique to imbibe these 'divine word energies', so that these get into her unborn's basic DNA and the memory system. The results were amazing. She gave birth to a healthy male baby, who is now three years old. And this child is called a miracle baby in their household. At this tender age, he uses high virtue energy words that he has never been taught. He receives love wherever he goes, all the kids long to play with him. He oozes ambience of love, compassion and sharing at this tender age, remains calm , peaceful and respectful.

Is this not a leader growing?

Oh yes, you bet!

I felt more motivated and socially responsible as I saw these miracle babies growing as distinct examples of the 'awakening in womb'.

The word *conception* is derived from *conceive,* meaning to create, to imagine, to invent a plan. It lies within your ability to create something extraordinary in your life by inventing a "grand plan."

Most of us are not aware of our power to create, imagine and plan our own invention. We leave it as a random act of growth, totally dependent on the environment, our uncontrolled, unmonitored thought patterns and emotions, that directly affect not only the growth of our baby, but also form the baby's future attitudes towards life.

MY SPIRITUAL GURU, MY UNBORN

How many of you have had, or are facing the problem of excessive vomiting? Especially in the first three months of your pregnancy ? (1st trimester)

- How many of you have felt weird mood alterations and have become choosy about food?
- How many of you have witnessed incidence of vaginal bleeding or spotting?

There are several physical, emotional and mental changes taking place, all simultaneously, inside all your bodies.

We in the present modern times, have somehow started dealing with pregnancy as something happening to us externally, like some pathology. We are so questioning (read fearful) of the course of pregnancy and the outcomes, that the first thing that we do is, "plan a visit to the doctor." It is alright to have yourself listed and started on the prophylactic regime. But as your visits grow by numbers, so does your fear, or may I put it, vice versa?

The moment we send our blood samples for screening of diseases and start gulping medicines for vomiting or for health, we somehow have already stepped into the zone of "FEAR" and being a "patient" :

- What, if something comes up in my blood reports?
- What, if I miss my daily tablets?
- What, if I start bleeding/spotting?
- How will I manage my work with pregnancy?
- What, if my husband does not take the responsibility that he should?

- What, if I am not capable enough of holding my baby?
- What, if I am not a good enough mother?
- These doubts and fears have already set in-- the first energy that has set in is that of "Fear/ Doubt".

Let's now have altogether a different point of view:

- What, if your new angel inside you is for your upliftment and growth?
- What, if your unborn is your protector?
- What, if your unborn is the energy which will bond you and your husband even stronger?
- What, if your unborn is there to empower you?

Doesn't all this bring courage, hope and joy to you?

Let us take this from another perspective altogether:

The very reason this pregnancy has happened at this point of time in your life means and reveals a lot about your current and future incidences. At this moment, be completely focused in the present and answer these questions. You may write them down :

- What is your current emotional state?
- How is your relationship with your partner?
- How is your financial situation?
- Mentally, how strong are you?
- Are there any physical problems, diseases that you are currently facing?

The first answer that has popped up is your most authentic answer. Don't analyze, just write them down with intuition.

If there is any problem in any sphere of your life, then this unborn has come to empower you, to give you hope and positive beliefs in that area of your life.

For example, there may some relationship issues between you two through your pregnancy. Won't the very thought of your incoming angel be able to re-establish or re-kindle that loving bond, to reignite that lost passion?

You will encounter challenges and situations until you work towards your relationship with a positive attitude, for a positive outcome!

If it is financial, you need to look at the core issues in your personality, your belief patterns and your beliefs around money. Take a journey into self and identify your financial patterns, your ups and downs. This new energy will help you not only in identifying this pattern, but even breaking it and transforming into a desired pattern. This is the time to take charge of your financial status and overcome all the pregnancy-related challenges.

This may sound a little baffling and "too much to digest", but this is it! There are no coincidences in life and so is with this pregnancy.

Pregnancies are a beautiful state of mind and life, where you are offered the opportunity to overcome a single or more chronic challenging patterns of your life.

If you are encountering emotional charges, imbalances in your life, this is the time to bond with your unborn with pure love and compassion and let go of any past emotional traumas, baggage and memories. This is the time to bask in the pure divine love with your unborn.

We are the logical and intelligent beings who have the power of "free will" of choice. Because of ignorance, beliefs and conditionings, we often let go of this spiritual opportunity, called pregnancy, consciously. So unfortunate, this !

The universe will work the way it does. Adversities and challenges will be faced in the areas where our empowerment is impending to be in. We will then have to undergo them experientially and learn. Generally, we miss this opportunity, of being simple and adapt. The higher purpose of this spiritual evolution is obvious and yet too remote.

For thousands of years, we as humans, have lived and experienced fear, separation, greed, competition and doubt. Now is the time to experience freedom, unison, cooperation, oneness, integration, total acceptance, compassion and finally the TRUTH.

This is also the time when the highly evolved souls (energies, fragments) are taking charge, creating the momentum. It is all in our highest interest and in the interest of all that we allow them to do that.

THE STORY OF NAMAN

In June 2015, Bharti, wife of Dharamveer, walked into my chamber. She was distressed, without hope and disappointed.

They had been married for 11 years now. She had been going through the turmoil of a strife-torn marriage, with a drinking, abusive and a straying husband. She had a son, 8 years of age, had lost a son after his birth. Both were caesarean operative deliveries at Agra. Their second son had died in his early days at nursery (with 8 month delivery). She had been transfused with multiple bottles of blood, was severely anemic and was cautioned of a dark future. Steeped in hopelessness, they faced very bad times ahead.

Another pregnancy, or a child, was a distant dream. She just wanted a revived relationship in her marriage.

She started attending the classes we offered. She began clearing her past, forgiving mostly, and after sometime, finally understood at the bottom level, that her husband was merely playing a role in her life, to help her make changes, letting go, embracing and empowering herself truly.

After the 5th class, she noticed that her relationship had improved. Her husband had apologized, returned to love her and completely stopped abusing. She was now living the blissful life of dreams.

But this was not the only thing to happen. The next week, she came to me with a smiling face. She said she had conceived after 6 years and against all odds. We both knew intuitively that there is no stopping and this baby is coming.

We crafted processes for her, did her the needed healing and alongside, put her on the contemporary, modern, supportive medicines. Although there were a few challenges during the entire course, nothing could deter us. Both her earlier babies were delivered at the 8th month of the pregnancy at 33-34 weeks of gestation, both had gone to the nursery, one had survived and the other had not.

Bharti carried this pregnancy right up to the middle of the 36th weeks in spite of the thinning scar of the previous caesareans. The caesarean was uneventful. The baby was healthy and did not need nursery support. She did not need any blood transfusion either!

The moment I had the baby in my lap (I knew he was not an ordinary soul). I felt like bowing to him and intuitively receive the messages he had for us. This was a highly evolved soul, no doubt about it!! Yes, she cleansed herself and allowed the highly evolved soul (HES) to use her womb as an instrument of wonderful creation of God.

Now, as I write, Naman is 6 months old. He can already sit, concentrate, laugh, demand, has an inclination towards chanting and can focus on the mantras of universal sound of "OM". He has never needed a diaper, as he has been indicating on his bowel, bladder evacuation needs. He is one of these miracle babies that we have been able to facilitate into this world through "cleansing, accepting and allowing."

But when I know, I just know it !
The fool will need the proof !

It is high time we understood that we, as parents, are only allowing the other soul to come to this world. We do not own them. We are their caretakers at the physical, emotional, mental and spiritual levels. The sooner we understand this, the better for us.

They are born with the wings, we just have to provide enough space for them to spread and take off.

How clutter-free we are at the physical level (disease-free), emotional level (strength of our emotions) and the mental level (our control over our thought patterns and awareness around our belief systems) to decide who will choose us as their parents.

This equation is as simple!

Mostly, we also have karmic relationships and karmic contracts. Karma works on the principle of cause and effect. Now imagine this, if by one's choice and willpower, we have switched our vibrations to a higher note, we will attract souls with whom we will nullify our karma of those vibrations.

Our give-and-take of one karma also depends upon the frequency at which we are vibrating. If we are at guilt, shame, jealousy, we will attract a soul who will teach us to be guilt-free, self-respecting and appreciating, by letting us experience more guilt, shame and jealousy, unless we experientially learn the opposite lesson. Sometimes, a lifetime is stuck with a simple, single lesson to be learnt with repeated patterns for the same lesson!

On the other hand, sometimes the progress is so quick that several lessons are accomplished in a short span of time, all depending upon the choices we make and the habits we form. We execute the courage and truth with which we live.

Be your highest truth, transform and let the light shine through you.

It is indeed in the highest of all good, to be able to manifest a genius, a world class leader, who has the potential to not only touch millions of lives, but also transform them!

PART 2

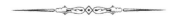

THE THREE TRIMESTERS

THE FIRST TRIMESTER

1st, 2nd, 3rd month

The blessings have showered and you are the one your baby has chosen to come through! You are perfect as a mother, father, a couple or a family for your child to be a part of. ☺

No one on this entire planet could have been pregnant with this baby, this energy! You have conceived at the divine time and you are blessed. You have allowed your body to be a channel for this energetic manifestation in the form of a baby, which will be formed by your own blood, tissues, emotions, thoughts and beliefs. This baby is so much a part of you, your own extension...it is separate and yet is not, it is you, whole and complete. You have embarked upon a journey of integration, not just with your child, your spouse, but most importantly, with the most important person in your life, YOURSELF!

Just for a while, close your eyes and visualize—imagining the entire global population, women who are pregnant just as you are at this given moment of time, millions of them and billions of permutations and combinations possible of partners coming together to have a baby. Your husband/partner is your perfect match amongst those million possibilities and that particular sperm of his, fertilized your ovum out of other millions! The chances of this particular baby, firstly coming through you and secondly coming to you both are infinitely less. All this is mind-boggling and yet you are blessed with this one "unique" energy-- your unborn, your baby now.

Could it be a random act?

Coincidence?

Or perfection?

Nothing in this life ever is a coincidence. All whom we meet, come across, strangers giving us smiles, places, cities and countries we visit, are never coincidences. All is aligned and in a perfect order, almost crafted. All this seems to be random and chaotic, yet there is always a perfect order. Our purpose behind the choices we make is also our guiding force with which we may be connected consciously with awareness or unconsciously in unawareness.

However, the fact is that things are as they were meant to be. This pregnancy too is not an exception. The synergy in the energetic system of you and your partner has accurately attracted your baby's energetic vibrations, most suitable for your own spiritual evolution. You will learn, unlearn, change and adapt as your pregnancy progresses and as your child grows after the birth. Your child will help you with your own enhancement in your journey, posing little challenges, and these challenges are your gifts, your pathways to improvement, to be the better and a higher version of yourself.

Accept this blessing wholeheartedly, with peace, calmness and gratitude, because you have no idea what you have harnessed as your baby, an infinite intelligence, is also your own guru for now. You have been given the responsibility as its creator, caretaker and protector.

This is the perfect time, and no time could have been any better. Repeat the following statement at least seven times with your eyes closed, NOW.

"I embrace change with ease and grace!"

The moment you allow yourself to create— even a single negative thought of fear, doubt, anger, rejection, shame, guilt, blame or complaint that you may feel, would be gone "off tangent" and because of your own free will and choices, you shall change and dictate the course of your pregnancy.

Let me dig a bit deeper here.

Being humans, how do we live? Through our free will and choices...correct? Yes, we do have a broader destiny plan, major event points that we shall touch, but the path and the course is absolutely our choice. The major lessons that we had chosen to learn and integrate in this lifetime, may sometimes take hundreds of lifetimes as we are so much stuck in the vicious cycle of give-and-take that most of the times our entire purpose of existence is lost. We succumb to diseases, miseries, self-pity, low self-esteem, hopelessness and start at even a lower destiny point in the next birth, lifetime or energetic evolution cycle.

God gave His power to the ignorant, the power was misused, misunderstood and ignorant we remained

Similarly, the entire period of nine months of the foetal life begins at day one of the conception and ends at the day last, the day on which the divine birth takes place.

Give yourself the permission to embark on this journey with your unborn.

One sperm out of millions fertilizes the ovum to form one cell (zygote) that inherits 23 sets of chromosomes from each parent, 46 in all. This is called conception. At this moment, the genetic make-up is complete, including the sex of the baby. Within about 3 days after conception, the fertilized egg divides itself very fast into many cells. It passes through the fallopian tubes into the uterus, where it attaches to the uterine wall, getting ready to be shaped into a tiny baby with very small hand buds, leg buds and the head along with the main torso.

The earliest changes you may observe in yourself at the physical level are the morning sickness, your appetite is rising and so is your tendency to throw up! You may get food craving too early during your pregnancy or notice that your favourite foods and drinks are suddenly unappetizing. Aversions to tea, coffee, milk and fried food are common among new mums to be. You suddenly develop liking for the weirdest foods.

I remember how I was craving for something like roasted potatoes and black salt, at 3.00 AM post-midnight, during my first pregnancy, giving a hard time to my husband, a resident doctor pursuing his post-graduation then. I had suddenly developed a strong affinity towards roasted potatoes with black salt! It seemed so crazy then and yet so perfect, my body was losing a lot of potassium as I was severely throwing up, almost two times every hour. My body was constantly dehydrated and was craving for potassium-rich food to replenish the loss.

Our body speaks to us. It knows how to heal itself. It is all about connecting with ourselves and following our own inner guidance. Roasted potatoes and black salt are good sources of potassium which is what my body needed and I was demanding exactly the same.

You, too, need to listen to your body. It demands what it needs. (Here you also have to distinguish between 'needs' and 'addictions'). You cannot fall for your addictions to the junk, disciplining self is the need of the hour here. Make a list of the food that your body is craving for, find out its nutritional value and treat yourself to some amazing, crave-satisfying food. You deserve this treat by all means .Believe me, you will feel divine and truly blessed, this is exactly what you need to indulge in!

Pregnancy hormones also have an effect on you, so don't be surprised if you feel tired and weepy. During the day you may feel tired and struggle to stay awake. Here, your body is preparing itself to support your baby.

All this is happening at the physical level. Do you have any control over it?

The answer is 'NO'. We cannot, although we have researched enough to discover the mechanism of evolution, forming and shaping up of the baby's body, including the physiology at work, but can we create this working mechanism in anyone? The answer again is NO. Our thinking logical mind is a minuscule of intelligence. It is the tiniest possible permeating part of LIFE!

THE FOUR BODIES

Let us come back to our four bodies that we discussed earlier. Any person on this planet primarily has four bodies-- physical body, mental body, emotional body, spiritual body-- and the 5th is the cosmic body, our higher self, our purest form of existence. For now, we are primarily going to focus on the four bodies and stay connected to our purest existence, our cosmic body.

PHYSICAL BODY
Your physical body is the one through which your spirituality, emotions and creativity flows. These are the vibrational fields of energy that overlap and affect each other profoundly. Our physical body is the ultimate ground where our thoughts and feelings manifest through actions and ultimately the results. Whatever we undergo emotionally, think mentally, surrender spiritually, is assimilated and shows up as a result on and through our physical body.

EMOTIONAL BODY
Your emotional body is the sum total of all the emotional experiences you've had so far. The word emotion means *"energy in motion"*, where thoughts and feelings go and the energy flows. Hurtful, fearful, angry and guilty—all kinds of emotions are held energetically as layers of memory. Therefore, if you have not healed your past traumas and emotional wounds, they sit as potential impending energetic discharges. The volcano erupts on the slightest trigger with these unhealed parts of the past and you remain mostly emotionally vulnerable. The loving, blissful moments have the soothing effect on the emotional body, these too create memories. This body has the most profound effect on your

unborn developing inside you. The emotional memories are carried through water and your blood, crossing the placental barrier and soaking your baby's system with both unconscious and conscious unhealed emotions.

MENTAL BODY

The divine mind is what majorly makes your mental body. A small part is also the egoistic mind, which drives you for your expanded awareness, motivates for achievements and fulfillment of various desires. The scenario though has reversed, of late, as the modern human has evolved. There is a loss of touch with the pure divine, powerful, manifesting mental body and the desire-driven egoistic mind has taken the driver's seat. Dominant, ego-driven thoughts, will lead to the passing of a mechanical, manipulating selfish mind from the mother to the baby, which is very weak, both mentally and emotionally. Meditation and inner connection is a simple way of letting your divine mind expand.

SPIRITUAL BODY

Our Spiritual body is activated when our physical, mental and emotional bodies are balanced and in harmony. The gateway to cosmic and infinite inner wisdom is opened, the inner light shines powerfully, and this becomes the state of instant manifestations in life. An activated spiritual body in the mother has the potential to attract the highly evolved soul of highest order, a future world leader, a great scientist, inventor, artist, world class singer, sports person , a very wise soul or a spiritual guru!

The first trimester (1st, 2nd, 3rd month) is the most crucial of the three, as the foundation of the entire body at the physical, chemical, biological, genetic and, most importantly, energetical level is laid out here.

The 3 developing germ layers (top, middle and third) carry the blueprint of this incoming human's existence. Multiplying exponentially, the cells have memories and codes full of encrypted information on the structure of the baby's body, how it shall unfold itself at the physical, mental and the physiological level blueprint to his internal organs, body structure, skin, hair, bones, muscles, all the organ systems, hormonal glands, the functioning of different cells, tissues, organs, organ systems and the functioning of the body as a complete single unit.

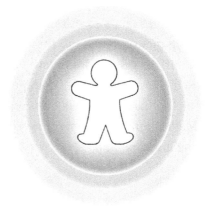

The four bodies: Physical, Emotional, Mental and Spiritual.

We, at the medicinal level and as clinicians deal primarily with the body structure and the functioning of the baby's body, often forgetting that the body is a mere vehicle to carry the driver, i.e., the energy of your baby. What is the energy of the baby going to be like? It's likes, dislikes, temperaments, reactions responses to challenging situations, attitudes, perceptions and the love, courage and kindness quotient. A few energetic blueprints are being created as you read this book . How about not just focusing on the physical body, (which is very important and cannot be ignored), but also on the real time, life-affecting aspects which are forming as the programmes on the basis of which your baby's life is going to run and re-run? These programmes and conditionings are the basis, the blueprints, depending on which your baby will make the choices in his/her life.

The interconnectivity and harmony of the body's entire biochemistry and functioning of all organic systems fundamentally fall into sync here: **WendellBerry**

WendellBerry

- What decides the final outcome?
- What decides the genetic expression?
- Is it all random?
- Is someone sitting up there and guiding the growth of the baby and the entire matrix of the human systems, cell by cell, tissue by tissue, organ by organ?

'HOW', is another question!

Barring just 1% of the genetic disorders, the baby's entire genetic expression, the entire body structuring is decided by YOU, your subconscious mind programming, your belief patterns and mental conditionings. *Yes, You Are "The" Power House.* You have invited this energy inside you and you are choosing everything, that may be, for your baby.

As Dr Bruce Lipton, a renowned cell biologist, writes in his book, **'The Biology of Belief'**: "The scientific premise has one major flaw— genes cannot turn themselves on or off. In more scientific terms, genes are not 'self-emergent', something in the environment has to trigger the gene activity."

At this juncture, it is important for our logical, reason-seeking minds to understand this completely, because this is the foundation of the very existence. Any doubt at this point may simply programme your unborn for the doubts at various levels. For me, DOUBT is,

D - Destroy
O - Outcomes
U - Unfolding
B - because of NO
T - Trust

Whenever there is a breach of trust, due to skepticism, separation and the fear of unknown, DOUBT crawls in. Doubt and suspicion are like small termite insects which cripple the existing human systems in form of individuals (self-doubt), families, societies and nations. Doubt, globally, is the number one source of inhibition, ignorance, fear, anxiety, below-average life, life full of unfulfilled desires and ultimately self-invited life of unfulfilled dreams.

I advise you now to quench your thirst completely. Explore the internet sites and gather all you can on epigenetics (if your mind still needs the scientific proof!). Or, you may choose to completely soak yourself in FAITH and start on this beautiful journey as it unfolds from here. If we are together on this, we proceed further, if not, you may put this book aside right away, as this is going to talk a lot about faith, belief and trust.

Epigenetics is a new type of science that is growing in popularity and promise in the scientific world. Epigenetics is the study of cellular and physiological traits, or the external and environmental factors that turn and define how our cells actually read those genes. It works to see the true potential of the human mind, and the cells in our body, says Dr Bruce Lipton. Eminent scientist, Sir Adrian Bird, and several others, are beginning to see the potential in this science.

It is understood that the environment is most important, same gene can *express* itself *"in more than 30,000 different ways, depending upon the different environments it is exposed to"*, says Dr Lipton, cell biologist, internationally recognized authority in bridging science and spirit. The worldwide researches show that genes and DNA do not control our biology; instead, *DNA is controlled by signals from outside the cell, including the energetic messages emanating from our positive and negative thoughts.*

Our environment functions at the two levels:

- Internal environment
- External environment

Our outer environment is a mirror reflection of our inner environment

Let me explain this a bit,

The prolonged, persistent experience of anger, fear, shame courage, compassion, passion and power in your internal environment has an effect to make these energies dominantly available to you, externally.

To change the experience in your outer environment, you must change the experience that you are having in your inner environment, your own inner self. Your inner environment is your unborn's external environment. Its growth--mental and emotional abilities, the physical features, organs and organ systems, IQ, EQ, SQ--are the result of the environment that it is growing in, and that is YOU! Here, you may refer to the experiment of Dr Masaru Emotos, a Japanese scientist, on the frozen water crystals that suggest that water has memory and our environment controls the result.

The root here is the THOUGHT.

For the highest good to manifest for your developing baby, the environment (both inner and outer), i.e. *you*, need to undergo change. Define the areas you want to improve upon and not pass it to your unborn. It could be in the areas of relationships, finance, health, spirituality, career and many more, that you have ident ified as limiting, un-serving or requiring a change.

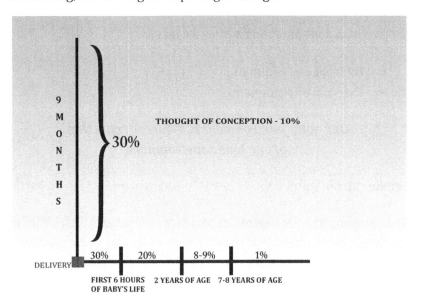

BLUEPRINTING THE SUB-CONSCIOUS MIND OF BABY.

EMBRACE YOUR POWER TO BLUEPRINT

Your baby's subconscious mind has been blueprinted, (future programming for life) on his relationships, emotional strengths, beliefs about families, marriage, finances, work, society, business, job, academics, trust, faith, anger, anxiety, love, courage, passion, compassion, happiness, joy, sorrow, sadness, etc. You have already blueprinted a 10%, starting with a thought, until the time you have conceived.

Rest of the 30% of blueprinting will take place in the upcoming 3 Trimesters.

Ist **Trimester** (1st, 2nd, 3rd month) = 10%
IInd **Trimester** (4th, 5th, 6th month) = 10%
IIIrd **Trimester** (7th, 8th, 9th month) = 10%

You will give what you have! Our conditionings are very strong and often we have little or no control over them, we innocently pass them over to our child. Rest of the 50% of your baby is blueprinted by the age of 2 yrs, rest 8 to 9 % by the age of 7 to 8 yrs, and after that it is 1% throughout the life.

There are three steps to blueprinting:

1. Become aware of our own conditions, belief systems and patterns.
2. Recognize the ones you would like to change for yourself (all un-serving and those blocking your own progress).
3. Break these patterns and create new serving ones and then pass it on to your kid.

All this work is easy, simple and could be achieved with a little effort. All you need to do is focus and connect with your subconscious mind.

How?

This could be achieved with awareness, affirming daily, until it becomes a ritual for you.

Daily Repeating Actions Become Our Rituals

And we are the product of our rituals or daily habits. It usually takes up to a minimum of 21 days and an average of 66 days for a habit to form.

For example:

If you are undergoing a major emotional turmoil in your life, or facing a major financial challenge, the beliefs you may have are:

1. Relationships are not **trust**worthy.
2. I cannot **trust** people with my money.
3. People backstab me.
4. Employees and bosses are there to take advantage.
5. There is a lot of injustice in the world, etc.
6. I am not lovable enough.
7. People are there to take advantage of me, etc.

This is the time to stop and understand that we are not BORN with these belief systems to be ours. These are the conditionings that we get from our parents, families and society in general.

After we adapt to these conditionings as our own, we start attracting situations that will deepen the pre-existing belief systems, as this is the exact energy that we are carrying inside us. We will encounter such experiences which will further deepen this pattern.

In between all this exists a brilliant goodness, that at this very moment you can CHOOSE, to let go of all these un-serving patterns and replace them by adopting the new, more serving ones.

Example:

1. Relationships are full of love and integrity.
2. I trust people with my money.
3. People around me are honest, fair and cooperative.
4. My working environment is harmonious, cooperative and joyful. There is a lot of support for me.
5. World is a beautiful and a peaceful place to be in.
6. I am lovable enough and I am loved.

The first month essentially is to focus upon your belief systems and replacing them. We dwell into stories our parents' experiences, our own experiences and make them the truths of our lives, which is far from the truth. No incidence is true or false, good or bad, it is all just an experience!

VISUALIZATION

Visualize this picture (of the three germ layer) daily while sending your love and saying:

'There is harmony and peace all around'

As I have said earlier, emotions are *"energy in motion"* and, therefore, any blocked, locked and withheld emotion will cause a diminished flow or stagnation in the flow of this energy , which causes delays, lack of motivation, diminished enthusiasm, various aches and pains and often disease as they grow dense when ignored.

Let us look at what is going on inside at the physical level, with the three germ layers forming the basic structure of a future well grown body. The neural tube (Brain, spinal cord and other neural tissue of the central nervous system) are developing.

The digestive tract and the sensory organs begin to develop. Bone starts to replace cartilage. The embryo begins to move, although the mother cannot yet feel it.

By the end of the second month, your baby, now a foetus, is about 2.54cm (1 inch) long, weight about 9.45gm. (1/3 ounce) and one third of the baby is now made up of head. Your baby's head may seem hugely larger than the rest of the body combined.

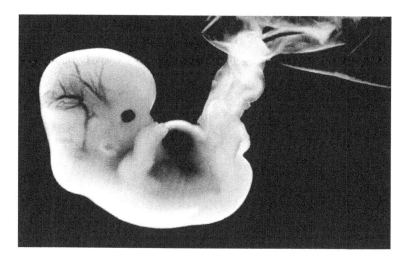

Brain is the fastest developing organ for now. Your baby is securely connected to you through the thin umbilical cord, which is its cord of HOPE and survival. All the nutrition, through your blood is reaching out to your baby and it is thriving on whatever you are supplying it with.

90% of the water, which is blood, is supplied to your baby through you, besides the vital nutrition, growth hormones and oxygen through blood. It also carries the energetic memories and memories that you have formed as a result of your experiences.

Yes, your baby is being offered experiences, memories, feelings and emotions, through you. 90% of your fetus's body is made up of water too. It floats like a fish in the vast 'pacific ocean' of its own, the water bag. The 'universe of survival' for your foetus is creating the basis of future programming inside the subconscious of your baby's mind already present.

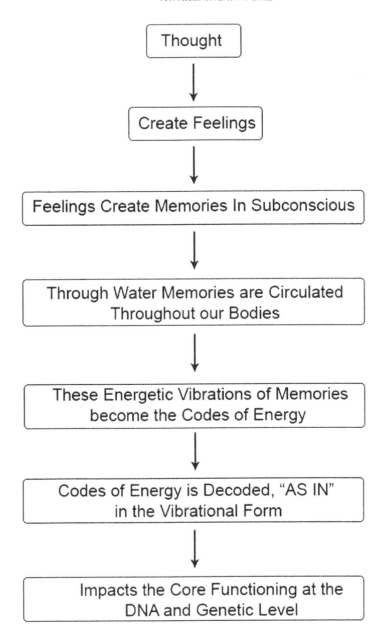

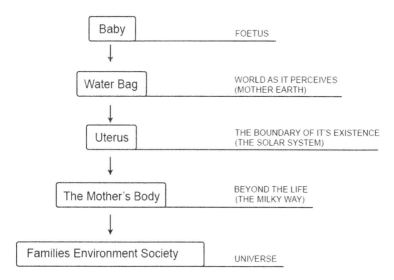

How do you relate to your planet, your existence in the solar system, in the galaxy and all of the universes that exist ? The chances are that we have not ever thought about it anytime, so far, it doesn't matter to us and by the way, why should we? How does it affect our *'beingness'* as individuals that we are?

Does the uterus, mother's body and the environment matter to the developing foetus? YES, not just matter, but the baby cannot survive without them . Just as you cannot survive without the solar system and the galaxy , but you have hardly even thought about it..

What is baby's perspective? Does it need only the planet (the water bag) for its survival? Can't the baby "FEEL" anything beyond it as of now?

Yes, this is also the time of "THE JUDGEMENT".

The initial vibrations that are received by the foetus are the vibrations that you are feeling right now, at the present moment.

Is it love, bliss, courage, and joy?

Or

Fear, uncertainty, doubt, anger, guilt, shame or even suspicion?

What energies are you supplying your foetus with?

Through my research for more than 15 years, I have discovered a lot. Similar to what Dr Thomas Verny and John Kelly have written extensively in the book: *"The Secret Life Of The Unborn Child". They write: "The unborn child is an aware, reacting human being who, after the 14th week, leads an active emotional life."*

"The foetus can hear, experience, taste and, at a primitive level, even learn in utero. What he discovered was that what the child feels and perceives begins shaping his attitudes and expectations about himself. What he ultimately sees himself and hence acts– happy or sad, aggressive or meek, secure or anxiety-ridden, all depends upon the messages he gets about himself in the womb."

"Deep persistent patterns of feelings, worry, doubt or anxiety that a woman carries rebound on her child. Chronic anxiety, notion about motherhood can leave a deep scar on an unborn child's personality. On the other hand joy, anticipation and elation contribute significantly to the growth of the child."

Dr Lester Sontang demonstrated in 1930's and 1940's that maternal attitudes and feelings could leave a permanent mark on the unborn child's personality.

This is also the moment to fully understand and totally remember that you are NOT the victim of your genes, genes which are powerful enough to modulate and affect the way they are going to be triggered and expressed, especially in the lives of our children.

And the "Biology of belief" says : The true power to regulate the genes lies with the environment the individual is in, the predominant thoughts, i.e, the true *power* of awareness, Identification, and replacement.

Anger and resentment are fire – not holy though. They will burn everything inside

The neurochemicals secreted as an affect of harboured anger and stress cause imbalance in the serene, sensitive hormonal balance axis that is necessary for nurturing the foetus. These neurochemicals create an adverse environment for the growth and survival of the foetus.

Thus, the altered hormonal axis may lead to:

- Missed abortions
- Spontaneous abortions
- Recurrent pregnancy losses (RPL)

Most women are intuitively in touch with the soul that is to be born through her (consciously or unconsciously). Some of the souls with difficult or challenging karmic interplay when conceived, give subconscious threat to the mother. It directly depends upon your mental, emotional state when you did conceive your baby. In feeling challenged, (you will eventually attract the soul corresponding to your vibration in your life at that time) subconscious threat comes to the mother. Consciously, they may not be aware and yet subconsciously they are anticipating rough times for the child.

Here, I would like to bring to your attention a very beautiful perspective which I have deduced after dealing with lakhs of patients over a period of little less than two decades.

The set of experiences of life, which a vibration brings to us, is unique.

For example,

If you are a very angry person in and out, you will continuously attract and invite anger in your life, including in the life of your incoming baby. However, it could also be in the highest likelihood, that through this unborn, you will learn to be at acceptance and peace and letting go of your anger as a lesson through your journey, as a result of the karmic contract between the you two.

On this journey, if you become aware of your anger issues and choose to resolve and dissolve them, it is in the highest likelihood that this baby, (whose contract with you is to impart lesson of peace and acceptance) may simply leave you or the contract may evolve with you to become a medium through which you may experience a whole new set vibrational emotions, i.e, your next level of lesson integration.

A possibility of converting your karmic relationship into a spiritual one is really high. This could be easily achieved by intention and acceptance.

THE CHALLENGES AND DISEASES THAT WE ATTRACT

Nausea and vomiting actually are indicative of a smooth running pregnancy, metaphorically have a deep energetic inference like past-life baggage, karmic lessons, etc. Pregnancy, being the time of energetic re-shuffling and re-alignment, all that we need to let go surfaces during this time and the body wants to throw up. This is a special time to pay close attention to your feelings. Here, it is important to observe, identify and heal yourself. What feeling is it, that is surfacing? Is it restlessness or irritation? Is it a feeling of burden or resistance? Or, are you feeling unfulfilled? Whatever it is, this is the time to completely accept and acknowledge and allow all the trash to go!

You may repeat to yourself,

> *"I assimilate and calibrate all the changes going inside my physical, mental, emotional and spiritual bodies. I flow, with the flow."*

Increased Mood Swings
Sometimes you may be full of zing and zest and sometimes lifting a finger becomes a chore. On some days you are cheery and chirpy, but on some you are queasy, essentially a gloomy belle. Hormonally, your estrogen and progesterone are playing with you and making you go for a ride.

Metaphorically:

It is the seesaw of getting to energetic compliance and balancing of the new energy that is growing inside you. This incoming energetic frequency, though, is at par with yours (after all, you have attracted it!) and is plus minus a few notches above or below you on the vibrational scale, but the adjustment of the environments is taking place. Your energetic system is adjusting with the new energetic system that you have recently invited.

It is like accepting, adjusting and going on the track, when you have guests staying over with you, for more than a while.

Bliss statement:

"I welcome my unborn and its set of new energies. I accept my new unborn as it is and invite acceptance from it. We both are in perfect harmony with each other."

Increasing Urge To Pee
Your visits to washroom are more frequent now. This too is related to hormones and the physical pressure of the growing size of the uterus on the urinary bladder, which is right beneath it.

Metaphorically:

Dr Masaru Emoto's experiment on the water, in the frozen form, shows that the words and emotions have deep memorial impact on the frozen water crystals. This corresponds to our body as it is more than 90% water. The initial memories of all kinds are, thus, deeply stored at the cellular levels in our bodies.

A lot of memorial baggage is shallowing up, during this period of alignment between you and your unborn. At the subconscious level, the processing of the memories is taking place. Water being the best carrier of memories, most of the un-aligned memories from the past/past lives, (where you both had been together earlier) not relevant to the present times, are discarded through frequent micturition, i.e, frequent passing of urine.

Food Cravings

Hormonal changes, coupled with a nutritional deficiency can lead to crazy food cravings from boiled potatoes to king-sized sliders. The list of food craving can go from bizarre to ridiculous. As long it doesn't harm you, it is alright to indulge in them.

Metaphorically:

One eats more as a compensation to one's past/ ancestral conditioning of LACK, scarcity and competition. The pregnancy is the result of culmination and intermingling of the three energies. A lot of past conditionings and past memories surface from the memory of struggle that one had during the early ages, struggling for food and survival. The tendency to eat more is the defence and protective mechanism against these surfacing past memories of PAUCITY and struggle. It is the by-product of the processing of the energies together.

The food (as water) also has an excellent memory bank-- energetically at the quantum level. The process of calibration of energies in its purest form is triggered by the memory system that water and food are carrying together.

The very earliest memories are triggered now and suddenly the craving for food starts and you are tempted to munch whatever you crave for and comes in handy.

Physically, by this time, your baby has grown up 2 cms in size. The tail of the embryo has begun to fade. Different nerve cells and muscle have started to function now. The baby's brain is starting to branch out and neurons have started to connect with each other. This is the beginning of creating neural pathways. The eyelids will be covering the entire eye now, fused. The formation of joints will begin. The wrist will see the small hand buds and the elbow move. The taste buds will start forming on your baby's tongue. Tiny earlobes have started to appear.

Visualize your tiny baby and send your unconditional love and support to it. This is the time of bonding and establishing energetic mutual understanding between the you two. Your somewhat natural statement at this stage may be:

'Oh my God ! I can't cope up with it any more. I am losing strength and I did not know that pregnancy is such a mess to be in.'

But a statement like this would potentially begin the relationship bonding between you two at the wrong note. This exactly is what is called the setting up of a karmic relationship with a lot of give-and-take accounts to follow in the future life between your baby and you.

CASE STUDY OF YASHODHA

Not long ago, October 2016, a very eager-looking couple, Yashodha and Gaurav came to me for guidance and assistance on conception. They wanted to have a baby, but were not able to conceive. Yashodha could not fully accept and adjust to the fact that she had to live with a new set of people after her marriage. She was mostly pleading to go back and stay with her parents. She was also dealing with her anger issues.

After an effective treatment, following identification and resolution of her core blockages, combined with contemporary medicinal support, she conceived soon. But still, she could not release her anger and resentment completely. My deeper study on her showed that her anger issues resulted in spotting and vaginal bleeding, posing a threat to the ongoing precious pregnancy.

We offered her counselling, emotional healing and strategies to deal with her anger issues, along with a strong hormonal support. Now, she was much relaxed, calmer and also began to accept her situation. But the off-and-on spotting was still an area of concern for us. I realized that medically and energetically, she was being offered all-possible support. So what it was that we were leaving out ?

Oh, we had not counselled the baby's energy !

After realizing the possibility of this gap, I took her for a session with her unborn. The thirteen weeks old foetus accepted the energetic healing and the counseling with the three of them-- Gaurav, Yashodha and this new incoming energy—went well.

Yashodha was willing to let go of her anger issues, and perhaps she realized, she no longer required these set of experiences. (her unborn was guiding her by challenging her through off-and-on vaginal bleeding. So, she completely accepted her anger and was much calmer now) What would be the baby's karmic contract with the would-be parents and for them to offer now? They asked and offered the baby to stay with them at a vibration of acceptance, love, peace and experience, accepting the new set of experiences that these new energetic vibrations would offer.

The bleeding completely ceased within 48 hours, her ultrasound report showed a healthy developing foetus of 13 weeks plus. And today, Gaurav and Yashodha are the blessed parents of a baby girl.

The law of free will and choices plays the most significant role in the process and outcome of a pregnancy.

Intentions and awareness matter too!

The lessons and learnings of a lifetime are not static and fixed. They are dynamic and changeable energetically. You are fully capable of raising your vibrations to higher levels than what your soul had planned initially before taking this particular birth.

Mind you, your children are our forefathers, lend your ear to them and they will load you with their wisdom..

A GODDESS CAN CREATE THE MAGIC OF A MIRACLE.

I am no less

-The mother

WELL BEGUN IS HALF DONE

The beauty of me is so gorgeous, that I am shining so within, so without.

Do you realize, you have actually allowed yourself to become the channel for divine's magic to play? You are the point of miracle creation.

- Who but the highest power can create life?
- Who are you?
- What is your potential?
- Are you any less than the God or the Goddess?

Find out for yourself.

This is the time to be in gratitude, for you have been made the medium to bring in a "MIRACLE". Also, to appreciate and acknowledge yourself as a powerful being who has an unlimited potential to create on an automated mode.

What was your first emotion, as you came to know about your incoming baby?

Was it a surprise?
Was it love?
Was it excitement?
Was it Hope?

Or

Was it nervousness?
Was it self-doubt?

Was it fear?
Was it complete acceptance?
Or, was it something else?

You exactly know the note at which your pregnancy has begun. How many of you had said,

"Oh my God! I can't have this baby, it is too soon.... Maybe, we can abort it."

Or

How many of you wanted this baby, but were not sure, as you felt the lack of support from your partner or your family?

Or

How many of you had "agreed" to get along, under the family's pressure?

Or

How many of you are filled with pure divine love, complete acceptance, and gratitude for the miracle to unfold and show itself?

Or

You have, somehow, conceived with artificial reproductive, assisting techniques, IUI/IVF and are now fearful, overwhelmed and non-trusting.

This I write with my experience of almost two decades. I've had women walk into my chamber with a variety of thoughts, feelings and emotions surrounding the news of their becoming mothers.

This energy shall sit as the basic foundation of energy inside your unborn, though still a tiny cluster of a few cells, as the three germ layers appear and start to expand. The mind and the consciousness the soul is, all knowing is already hanging around.

This, 'already existing' will be hidden after a few hours of birth as these memories will be shielded, including the programmes which have been written, are being written, and will be written. These programmes begin to be written with the first thought of conception and continue until the baby is delivered and is a few hours old. By this time, your baby has already been blueprinted approximately 70% with the programmes and conditionings which are going to guide and run nearly his entire lifetime or until the time your child becomes self-aware and decides to let go of these un-serving patterns and decides to adopt new ones, which he may realize experientially after observing his life unfold on limited thought processes and conditionings !(if at all, he realizes !!)

We may save ourselves from the guilt trip here, as we also blueprint our baby with the necessary life-saving, relevant, evolutionary programmes, natural instincts and desires which are necessary for the survival and progression. While we do so, our ego, fears and doubts, skepticism, shame, guilt, envy, anger, frustration and many more vibrations creep in, silently, innocently and unconsciously.

Reversing, and filtering all this is absolutely simple. All you need is to be highly aware of your current thoughts and thought patterns and see who you really want your baby to be. You will know all that, intuitively.

As the old saying goes, "Well begun is half done."

The difference here is that each moment is the new beginning. You really don't need to think or dwell in the past. Past has happened, and it is a powerless history. All the power that the past may have over you is being sucked from your present. It's time you made peace with your past, so completely accept it and render it powerless over your present. This is a choice you have NOW, right at this moment.

Letting go completely, dancing to the rhythm of life, flowing with it, will let you glow so much in, and so much out. Ok, let me ask you something here:

Do you consciously help form the organs of the baby?

Are you in any position to logically/ consciously develop, help or grow your baby, or any of his/her organs?

The answer, of course, is a big NO.

What options do you have, but to surrender and completely accept the magic at play, for the marvel of the creation's magic to unfold?

What you, as others, do is pose roadblocks by trying to control and navigate the flow of the pregnancy.

Your unborn, that tiniest baby, just a cluster of few cells barely has the heart beating at 6 weeks, is seen as a linear line fluctuation at live sonography, is actually your GURU already. Further into its growth, it will teach you and make you realize the most profound lessons of your life:

To appreciate the power of **surrender**, embrace the power of **complete acceptance**, the power of **allowance** and the power of **expectation.**

All you can do, and have to do, is just to ALLOW and say your sacred YES to the life. And truly speaking, you really don't have any more options beyond it.

What else you have other than this is:

The power to destroy it,

The power to sabotage its growth,

And the power to threaten the pulsating life itself.

Beside these negations, you and I can't do much to enhance the miracle of life that is growing inside you. Therefore, all we can do is to ALLOW and accept it !

Only if we could keep all our destructive, destroying, negating, contracting doubts and fears away from this, we have done our jobs. We have allowed and given our permission for the life-form to expand and BE.

The foremost point to be taken into consideration is the balancing of the energies. I have explained the *gunas* in detail in the Cosmic Conception, we need to raise the *sattva guna* to the maximum possible and properly balance the *rajas* and the *tamas gunas*, or the tendencies.

Just say, *"I allow and accept the divine life force to take shape and thrive inside me'*

We traditionally as a society have been advised on certain dos and don'ts during the First Trimester. Just sample a few of them:

- Not to travel far.
- Not to eat outside food.

- Not to watch horror movies or read such novels.
- To read our great scriptures and "good books."
- To avoid certain foods, even homemade ones!
- To consume daily good amount of water of good quality and so much more..

How relevant and scientific all these traditions are? Yes, our ancient rituals and guiding systems are not bizarre or random, in fact they are mostly scientific and logical. Travelling and eating outside food will expose you to different and a variety of foreign energies. At the assimilation point, how can you attract an intermingling bunch of confusing energies leading to mixed and confused thoughts? At this crucial time, how can a confused programming and conditioning be allowed to happen to the subconscious of your growing baby? You may pause here, take a few deep breaths and rest for a while and think,

Are you there to cause uncalled for disruption in the life of your growing baby?

ENERGY IS EVERYTHING AND EVERYTHING IS ENERGY

The outside, market-prepared has the energetic content of the ingredients, of the people cooking it, intention and mood of the people involved in the preparation of that food. First Trimester is essentially a period of mega conversion of high potential and kinetic energies of the egg and sperm to a billion celled multi-cellular organism, i.e., your baby's initial body. And here, you want an intervention which is foreign to your unborn's energies. Why?

Mind you, this is the period of "assimilation and conversion."

All the energies that the mother's systems (physical, mental and emotional) are exposed to, are conversed, culminated and transitioned to the baby's body. All that you eat and feed yourself with, is forming and shaping your unborn's body.

Just see, how this is the period of pure transition of energy:

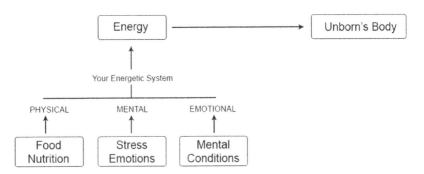

Whatever you eat and feed your body with, will transform into the body, brain structure, functioning and thinking in the conscious and subconscious mind of your unborn. The nutrition plays a significant role in building up your baby.

"Our food should be our medicine and our medicine should be our food."
– Hippocrates

"Your diet is a bank account. Good food choices are good investments."
-Bethenny Frankel

FOOD AND NUTRITION

Natural folates, natural phytogens, betaine, choline, and methyl rich foods are important in not just bringing about the balance in the vital important cycle in your body, but also a perfect genetic D.N.A structuring and restructuring. These are involved in epigenetic modification of your unborn. Folates (Folic acid) are the catalyst in synthesis and help in execution of various biochemical constructive cycles which are going on at the core D.N.A. levels.

Table of food for First Trimester:

Folate-rich foods : These should be consumed especially in the first trimester, as folates enhance the neural growth and prevent any neural defects in the incoming baby. Asparagus, broccoli, dark leafy greens, citrus fruits, papaya, oranges, grape fruit, strawberries, beans , peas, lentils, kidney beans, split beans, avocado, sprouts and nuts, sunflower seeds, peanuts, flax seeds, almonds, cauliflower, beets, corn, celery and carrots.

Vitamin B-rich foods: Few of the vitamin B-rich foods are oats, bananas, potatoes, avocados, kidney beans, summer squash, spinach, almonds and milk,

Betaine-rich foods: Wheat bran, beets, spinach, Amarnath grain, quinoa. Betaine is an amino acid that has potential benefits for fighting heart disease, improving body composition and helping promote muscle gain.

Choline-rich foods: Raw cauliflower, mushrooms cooked, dark promote-chocolate, leafy greens, beet greens cooked, asparagus, cooked cabbage, brussels sprouts, cooked bok choy (Chinese cabbage). Choline is the precursor to betaine. Foods rich in betaine are generally rich in choline.

Methyl-rich foods: All foods rich in vitamin B9 are folate-rich, including strawberries, citrus fruits and leafy vegetables, milk, toasted wheat germ, brussels, sprouts, broccoli, and all folate-rich foods.

A week's plan may look like:

A Week's plan may look like:

MONDAY				
BREAKFAST	**SNACK**	**LUNCH**	**SNACK**	**DINNER**
Porridge made with milk flavoured with a pinch of cinnamon & a tbsp apple puree Glass of apple juice	Yoghurt drink Orange	avocado salad Banana cooked kidney beans brown bread	Small fruit or cheese scone	peas, split beans or gram with brown rice

TUESDAY				
BREAKFAST	**SNACK**	**LUNCH**	**SNACK**	**DINNER**
Greek yoghurt and ginger with chopped fresh fruit (mango, peach or nectarine) served on pancakes Fruit smoothie	any citrus fruit puree Nuts , soaked almonds	Baked potato and cottage cheese Small bunch of grapes	Handful of dried apricots	Deep leafy greens with sprouted wheat wheat bran rich bread or chapaties

WEDNESDAY

BREAKFAST	SNACK	LUNCH	SNACK	DINNER
Bran flakes with semi-skimmed milk and sliced banana Glass of cranberry juice	Vegetable pancake	Broccoli and pea soup with a crusty roll Apple	Carrot sticks and hummus dip	Healthier green soup and apple casserole

THURSDAY

BREAKFAST	SNACK	LUNCH	SNACK	DINNER
Porridge made with milk flavoured with a tbsp of tinned berries in fruit juice. Green or herbal tea	Pot of low fat Yoghurt and Mango	Feta salad couscous Papaya	Slice of banana bread	Creamy mixed vegetable soup with asparagus and raw tenderly steamed cauliflower with a few seasonings

FRIDAY

BREAKFAST	SNACK	LUNCH	SNACK	DINNER
Wholegrain toast spread with peanut butter Yoghurt drink	Rice pot	Cranberry and soft cheese wrap with watercress Slice of melon	Breadsticks with low-fat soft cheese dip	Baked potatoes, broccoli and peas

SATURDAY				
BREAKFAST	**SNACK**	**LUNCH**	**SNACK**	**DINNER**
Greek yoghurt and ginger mixed with tbsp chopped dried fruit (apricots, figs or dates) and tbsp muesli Glass of orange juice	Small roll with peanut butter	watercress salad Kiwi fruit	2 fig rolls	Pasta with low-fat garlic bread

SUNDAY				
BREAKFAST	**SNACK**	**LUNCH**	**SNACK**	**DINNER**
cabbage and asparagus on toasted wheat bread Yoghurt drink	Banana	roast peas, cauliflower roast potatoes, **broccoli** and carrots Apple and pear crumble	1-2 handfuls of mixed nuts and dried fruit	Tofu and butternut squash flan

Any impure energies in the form of food hold a potential hazard to disrupt and bring about several undesired tampering with the sensitive and important changes taking place inside your body.

Consider this example:

Imagine, you are to construct the house of your dreams and you are laying the foundation. You would only want to put the best quality bricks, cement and other construction material. You will not allow the impurities to be added to the cement, since it will cause a weak foundation, in strength and structure. After all, this foundation will have to bear the load of the entire structure to be raised over it!

Any deviation from food, thought and energy can weaken the foundation laying in the First Trimester and affect the following :

1. Body shape of the unborn.
2. Energetic system of the foetus.
3. Distribution of energy throughout this tiny existing creature.
4. The most vital organ, BRAIN (inclusive of the MIND) which is acquiring shape and forming at a rapid speed.

The other most destructive energies, beside undesired food, are:

- ANGER
- FEAR
- DOUBT
- GUILT
- SHAME

These are the lowest and the densest vibrations that adversely impact the developing foetus.

I have discussed these energies, in detail, their impact on the incoming baby and have explained the effects they carry on the organs and the organ system, in the **forthcoming book** in this series.

It is my humble way of creating awareness about the powers we hold that disrupt the working ways of the universe, all because of our choices and free will. It is, therefore, important on how best and willfully we can assist the automated system to function at its peak?

For now, at this stage, you exactly know how you are in a position to only ALLOW the universe to perform at peak, by supporting it, with:

Good Nutrition, Food, And Positive Thought Forms

NO human on this planet is capable or is enough to consciously and logically understand the system of unfolding of a two-cell structure to a multicellular baby, leave alone creating it. *THIS IS AUTOMATED* and thank GOD it is automated and beyond human comprehension. Just imagine what humans would have done to the evolution of a baby inside the mother's body if they even knew an iota of the equation and understood the process and miracle of the making of a body of any species, what to talk of a human body. Each one so unique, each one a master piece, one of its kind! I may sound a bit snide and unkind, but I am sorry to say that if we had our way, with our conscious intervention (if we could, as we mostly strive), we would have been a horrid, disrupted human race today!

"Our scientific power has outrun our spiritual power. We have guided missiles and misguided men."
--Martin Luther King

We just have to look around ourselves through our cities, states, nations and our planet, to see the impact of human activities. *Conscious Evolution*, not blessed by **Nature**, brings destruction rather than construction around us, not just in the physical form, but in our minds and emotions as well.

An appeal to you, my goddesses carrying babies inside you: realize that you are unique, the chosen one and perfect for this baby. Please **allow** the universe to work its way to creating miracles as your babies. I request you all not to use your destructive powers (both consciously and unconsciously) on yourselves and your incoming babies.

"With Awareness, We Change."

Third thing which plays a very vital role in the foundation laying is water. Water has memory and memories create changes in the shape and alignment of the water molecules. The memories (both good and bad) translate to a deep effect on the functioning of the basic unit of life the CELL (as most of the content of the cells, tissues, organs, systems, blood and our bodies is water).

So, whatever we are, we are the results of our thought processes and beliefs. It goes on something like this:

Some stunning scientific discoveries about the biochemical effects of the brain's functioning show that the cells of human body are immensely affected by thoughts.

As Dr Lipton writes: "I came to the conclusion that we are not victims of our genes, but masters of our fates, able to create lives overflowing with peace, happiness and love."

An impressive body of research is documenting how important parents' attitudes are in the development of the foetus.

Dr Thomas Verney, a pioneer in the field of prenatal and perinatal psychiatry writes, "In fact, the great weight of the scientific evidence that has emerged over the last decade demands that we re-evaluate the mental and emotional abilities of unborn children. Awake or asleep, the studies show, the unborn is constantly turned into their mother's every action, thought and feeling. From the moment of conception, the experience in the womb shapes the brain and lays the groundwork for personality, emotional temperament and the power of higher thoughts."

This is also the time to realize that his concept of new biology is not a blaming agenda for mothers for every ailment that medicine didn't understand—from schizophrenia to autism. We need to understand that the conception happens with the culmination of energies of both mother and father. Father is equally responsible. Definitely, there are developmental hazards when the fathers leave their wives, or partners alone, or if the mother is facing abandonment emotionally, socially or economically. This definitely will contribute to the basic personality formation of the would-be adult.

A mother's thought is directly responsible for the unborn's growth and basic blueprint of it's subconscious mind. We need to clearly understand and mark the role that the father and members of the family play on the mental, emotional, spiritual and psychic health of the mother.

IF A MAN DESIRES TO BE THE FATHER OF AN EMOTIONALLY, PHYSICALLY AND MENTALLY STRONG BABY, HE NEEDS TO LOVE THE MOTHER UNCONDITIONALLY AND SUPPORT HER EMOTIONALLY, PHYSICALLY AND MENTALLY.

The masculine energy of the father is like a strong armour of support to the warm, intuitive and healing energies of the mother. A perfect balance and integration of the two will see through to a happy, healthy and a genius on its way!

"A mother full of Courage and Faith, coated with unconditional love, joy and peace will bring about a baby, a genius, a future world leader, who will hold the potential to change the course of humanity forever."

THE STORY OF SHAHANA

Shahana, a 30-year-old, well-built standing-tall female, had been through the trauma of several miscarriages, 6 to be precise. In medical terminology, this is called a case of Recurrent Pregnancy Loss (RPL).

In her way to the seventh pregnancy at seven weeks and three days, she lost all hopes. Shahana entered my chamber in the cold month of January. She was under medical treatment elsewhere, fully supported by all possible medicines in the form of oral and injectables that can be given to a RPL patient. She was suspecting a loss again and had come for an ultrasound scan and a second opinion. The ultrasound scan showed a perfect heartbeat of the baby with a little collected blood inside. After reassuring and adding a few more medication, she calmed down a bit, but only to return after minutes, howling and crying. Her bleeding was a full flow now as she sobbed inconsolably, wanting a D&C (Dilatation and curratage procedure to clean up the uterus), as she deeply felt that either she had aborted the baby or was on such a course yet again.

I suggested a re-scan to confirm if actually the baby was gone. To my relief and her amazement, the heartbeat of the baby was rhythmic and beating, though the blood collection had increased.

I took control of the situation. My "intuitive healer" sprang into action and soon I traced a strong suppressed anger, almost rage, inside her. She had been suppressing her anger forever and the rage was boiling inside her skin. Her family members were clueless. According to them she was very calm, peaceful and docile.

I had an intense two-hour long session with her. She created an awareness for herself, of what her anger was doing to her and her babies and that she was living in the vibrations of victim consciousness. The moment she released them and raised her vibrations, her face lit up with shine and hope.

That was the last day she saw herself bleed. The pregnancy progressed uneventful, full of hope and promise. She realized that whatever was happening in her life was created by herself. She had the power she could use to her benefit. Thus, she had become the power creator of her own life.

As Shahana regained awareness control over her life, realizing her potential to create anything and everything, all of you beloved mother are the true source of light. You are absolutely enough to change and transform your life in whichever direction you wish to!

Embrace and initiate your power within, the time has arrived.

CONCLUSION: Your anger, frustration, anxiety and fear can cause an unimaginable damage to your ongoing pregnancy. Recurrent bleeding issues, recurrent pregnancy loss or RPL may be due to the stored anger. *FEAR* is the vibration which leads to a 'missed' or a spontaneous abortion. These two are the energetic vibrations that you need to stay clear off, if unhealed you need to release these negative discharge which may be fatal to your unborn. Many cases of RPL, bleeding issues and of threatened abortions are dealt with very easily, effortlessly and efficiently with self-correction and awareness. We do it very frequently at our counseling sessions and during the workshops.

THE SECOND TRIMESTER

4TH, 5TH, 6TH MONTH

Second trimester is essentially the "BRIDGE" between you and the "just a few cellular tiny clusters to the would-be trillion cells" being. This bridge is transient, but plays the most important role in the subconscious mind programmes of your unborn which are to run it's future life .

The consciousness of the unborn is pure and expanded, the mind absorbs very quickly, eagerly, without any filters/filtrations of the cognitive/conscious mind.

The conscious mind is immersed in the subconscious. The unborn's conscious mind is the part of the subconscious with no filters and no boundaries. All that is subconscious is the conscious.

Baby's ability to comprehend, taste and hear is now well established and developing. The brain that has developed well has taken the shape and is still developing, the logical, cognitive "thinking" analysis is absent though. The mind of an unborn can be imagined as an enormous huge, dehydrated sponge kept in a pool of water. It absorbs and fills itself completely. The subconscious mind of the baby is eager, excited and ready to be filled with information, instructions, feelings, images that are projected to 'the' foetus through collective beliefs, conditionings, feelings, emotional states of the parents, family and the environment.

Maximum blueprinting storing of the belief patterns and conditionings is happening to your unborn now. Even as you read this, you may experience thoughts like:

I am not loved.

I am unsupported.

This pregnancy is troublesome.

What is going to happen?

How will things shape up?

My husband/ wife is so irresponsible.

Only if we had a little more money.

If only we had a better jobs and little more security.

If my family and husband could understand what am I going through... and so on.

Of course, not all of you will have all of these challenging thought forms, you may have most of these, a few of these, or if you are truly the blessed mom, none of these. I would also like to admit that not even once in my practice of 18 years, have I come across a single mom who has not had either of these innocent thoughts as concerns, which are now becoming the firm belief systems of the developing child inside her!

All these concerns have a root in the doubts and all these doubts shoot up from one or the other kind of fear.

Fear of future

Fear of failure

Fear of being judged, etc.

Fear is a crippling emotion. I will not say you need to "rise above" your fears. That will not help you. It will keep pulling you down! The best thing here would be to completely embrace all your fears and all your doubts. Say to yourself :

"I ACCEPT MY FEAR AND DOUBTS OF THE FUTURE OF THIS PREGNANCY. I ACCEPT THAT I FEEL UNSUPPORTED, UNCARED FOR."

The moment you start accepting things, things begin to change. This very moment, remember what you RESIST will PERSIST, what you accept will change.

Change is the very essence and compelling sign of life. Let the change begin by accepting, embracing and appreciating all that is "AS IS".

You not only do wonders to yourself, but also provide a base platform of acceptance as a belief in your developing baby. His core vibration has now shifted from doubt and fear to acceptance and appreciation.

You must remember that the baby still doesn't have a word bank, though s/he is absorbing your vocabulary and is most influenced by your feelings.

"FEELINGS ARE THE LANGUAGE OF THE SOUL"
– CWG

What your baby understands perfectly are the feelings that you are feeling. The feelings are thought-oriented. You cannot mask or shield your feelings, but you can genuinely have the more appropriate ones by examining your thoughts and thought forms.

Completely surrendering and operating with faith will see you through.

Slowly, you will see that by acceptance and appreciation, your perceived environment is also changed. You are the creator and the most important person in your life. You attract who you are. When you start appreciating all that, you start experiencing change and a shift in how things are in your environment.

This is also the best time to inculcate the belief of a healthy, beautiful body of yourself.

And why the belief of self like ?:

"Oh my God, how shapeless I have become, how fat, bloated and ugly I look. I have become so unattractive!"

Or

I am getting so much anxiety. My BP is either so high or so low, my feet are so swelled up, I am eating so much, oh God, what is happening to my body?

And so many more of these !

As your baby inside is absorbing all that you are feeling, you know exactly what are you blueprinting your baby with, what self-image, self-worth and self-esteem..

When you feel yourself being unattractive due to your pregnancy, there are three things entering your baby's subconscious:

- The pregnancy leads to my mom being unattractive (GUILT)
- Low self-image and self-esteem

- An option and a choice that a human body CAN be unattractive too!!

From the perception of the Creator, all His creations, including you, are unique, perfect and an epitome of beauty. For the Creator, the physical appearance is only a mere small portion of the endlessly beautiful WHOLE creation that you are!

Physical unattractiveness does not even exist as a choice. It is our mind's perception and belief of beauty and ugliness that creates that point of view.

As you enter your Second Trimester, start visualizing your baby from its head to the toe, visualizing, connecting with all his body parts, visualizing them function in rhythm and sync. This is also the time to send over health- energy, unconditional love to your unborn. Soon, your own thoughts will fill up with all positivity and HOPE, and you will start saying :

I SEND MY HEALING ENERGIES AND UNCONDITIONAL LOVE FOR A THRIVING HEALTH AND A PERFECTLY FUNCTIONING BODY OF MY BABY.

When you speak this to your baby, full of love and feelings, you are cementing him with securities for this life time and, GOD knows, many more to come!

I will not go into the details of organ and systemic development of your baby, nor am I touching upon the diseases that your child may get through you at these developmental stages. For now, my humble request to you is to understand that,

WHATEVER YOU FOCUS ON, EXPANDS

Rather than focusing on complications, diseases of the Second Trimester, focus on the well-being, health, beauty and wellness. Nutrition, your own stress and emotional feelings, have a lot to blueprint your baby with.

The word stress has taken a prominent position and place in our language worldwide. It expands to:

S - So much
T - Tension
R - Reserved
E - Emotionally
S - Situationally in
S - Subconscious Mind

This word has been given an undue importance and weightage. It has a potential hazard to attract doubt, fear, load, chaos, and burden in our lives.

Drop the word STRESS from your lingo right NOW.

This energy is highly un-serving and I can't emphasize enough, that this single word has the potential to burden and brings heaviness to your life.

On the other hand, pick up the word **challenge,** which is much better-- it is adventurous and fills you with a sense of achievement when met.

Andrea Garden so beautifully has said:

"CHANGE YOUR WORDS, CHANGE YOUR WORLD."

How and what you speak to yourself, forms the basic structure of the vocabulary of your incoming baby. Sentences innocently uttered, like "I am such an idiot", seem to be harmless or even cute, but these are immensely damaging to the psyche of your unborn.

FOOD AND NUTRITION

Not only physical, but also energetic growth of the fetus is affected both by the quantity and quality of the food you eat. Let me explain my perspective: If we go back to how the human race has evolved over thousands of years, we would know, that it was the need of the cave men to survive on the animal flesh, kill, eat and live. The bodies of these early men were huge and the intellect- intuition was minimally existent. As the evolution went by, plantations and agriculture evolved, the physical body changed in size, shape and structure. The intelligence and the intuition started coming into existence. What would the energy of a dying animal be? That of Fear? Struggle? Anger? Hopelessness? What energies will be harnessed through this dead animal's flesh? As we all know, this basic law of energy states,

Energy cannot be created or destroyed. It can only be transformed from one form to another.

You certainly would not want the energies of fear and aggression to enter your and your unborn's system.

There is a Hindi saying:

'jaisa khaoge ann, vaisa hoga mann'
(what you eat is what your mind is)

Switching to vegetarian diet is a good idea of the hour. We need lighter and higher vibrations, not the lower and denser ones for our intellectual, intuitive, creative and energetic growth.

You certainly need high protein diet, carbohydrates and fats to be taken in the right proportion. You already know a lot about your nutrition and have enough access to the information.

FATS are especially important for intake in the Second Trimester. Fatty acids are vital for the hormonal balance and growth of the foetus. Nuts have to be included extensively to your diet.

Table of diet schedule in the Second Trimester could be something like this,

Eat plenty of foods that help your unborn baby grow. Foods rich in omega 3 fatty acids will help your baby's brain development.

Calcium and vitamin D are essential for the growth of strong bones and teeth.

You'll need to have plenty of iron-rich foods. Iron helps make red blood cells for your growing baby.

Tip: don't drink tea or coffee with a meal – it makes it harder for your baby to absorb iron.

A Week's meal could look something like this,

MONDAY

BREAKFAST	SNACK	LUNCH	SNACK	DINNER
Porridge made with milk flavoured with a pinch of cinnamon and a tbsp apple puree Apple juice	Handful each of dried apricots and almonds	Super Salad Chopped papaya	Small fruit or cheese scone with spread	Chicken/cottage cheese and mushroom risotto Side salad

TUESDAY

BREAKFAST	SNACK	LUNCH	SNACK	DINNER
Pot of plain fromage frais mixed with chopped fresh fruit (mango, peach or nectarine) and a tbsp flaked almonds served on scotch pancakes Papaya smoothie	Sesame seed bar (good source of iron too)	Pistachio chicken with chopped mixed salad or smoked chicken and avocado salad Chopped pineapple	Hummus with pitta	Cottage cheese with pine nuts, broccoli and sweet potato mash

WEDNESDAY

BREAKFAST	SNACK	LUNCH	SNACK	DINNER
Wheat bisk cereal with milk with meshed/ sliced banana Papaya Smoothie	Pot of fromage frais	Watercress and celeriac soup with wholegrain toast and spread	Oaty cranberry and orange cookie	Spaghettli carbonara Wilted spinach

THURSDAY

BREAKFAST	SNACK	LUNCH	SNACK	DINNER
Porridge made with milk flavoured with A tbsp of berry compote Herbal tea	Fruit scone with spread	Sardines (good source of omega 3, calcium & vitamin D) on toast	Rye crackers with soft cheese	pie with carrot

FRIDAY

BREAKFAST	SNACK	LUNCH	SNACK	DINNER
Wholegrain toast spread with peanut butter Yoghurt Drink	Banana	Ciabatta with Halloumi basil and sundried tomatoes Orange	Slice of gingerbread	Kidney beans with tomatoes

SATURDAY

BREAKFAST	SNACK	LUNCH	SNACK	DINNER
Pot of Greek yoghurt mixed with tbsp chopped dried fruit, flaked almonds and tbsp muesli (make the night before and keep in the fridge of soften) Orange juice	Apple and bran muffin	Cheesy baked beans in a baked Potato	2 handfuls of walnuts and dried fruit	Stir fry soya nuggets with spring greens and noodles

SUNDAY				
BREAKFAST	**SNACK**	**LUNCH**	**SNACK**	**SNACK**
Scrambled eggs on toasted bagel with spread Yoghurt Drink	Rice pot	Sweet apple veggie Couscous And broccoli	Oaty cranberry and orange cookie	Mushroom and celery pasta bake

As I said earlier, the Second Trimester is bridging the First and the Third Trimester. It is supposed to be the easiest going and uneventful of the three and it is not surprising that the maximum blueprinting and conditionings happen around:

- Self-image, self-esteem
- Confidence
- Anger and aggression
- Viewpoints towards relationships, marriage
- Role of a mother and father
- General perception of the society and the world around
- Perceptions towards finances, business and economy
- Tendency for suppression or openness

And many more.

These basic belief patterns and the subconscious mind imprints formed in your unborn are going to run his/ her future life.

This is also the time when the *"Fetal genius quotient"* (FGQ) is shaping up. The FGQ is directly impacted and influenced by your own IQ ,EQ, SQ (intelligence, emotional and spiritual Quotients).

It is also a very good time to become aware of your own EQ, SQ, and IQ as these form the basis of the FGQ. Whilst you can't do much with your IQ, ☺ you certainly can do wonders with your raised EQ and SQ. As I often say during my workshops that our unborn is our *guru* through whom we learn and unlearn so much!

This is a beautiful time to come face-to-face with your own emotional strengths, weaknesses, sabotages and to raise your emotional vibrations to unconditional love, peace and kindness. Love is the basic emotion, which has the potential to conquer all the lower EQ and diminishing vibrations. Therefore, EQ with unconditional love, appreciation and acceptance of your OWN SELF is vital. And why not? You are the most beautiful, unique creation of God!

If you are not appreciative of the God's child that you are, how in the world you imagine yourself to be appreciative of your child, who is also God's creation, but through you !

Rage and anger issues at this stage have a potential to reduce (burn) the liquor (water in the water bag) in the Third Trimester. Mothers with such issues are often seen dealing also with the bleeding problem. Anger and rage may lead to lowering of the Amniotic Fluid Index (AFI). Suppressed anger often causes spotting and vaginal bleeding.

Chronic guilt, shame, emotional and financial insecurities may land your baby into Intra-Uterine Growth Retardation(IUGR). The guilt and shame form the basis of anger, especially suppressed anger. So, often IUGR is seen alongside oligohydranmios (reduction in the amount of water in the water bag).

My own observation during my long years of practice and research, clearly suggest that the lower vibrational frequencies and their emotional manifestations lead to a diminished inflow and hindered circulation of the cosmic life force, the **PRANA**, which is the basic, vital force of life.

The lower energies, when become denser, take shape of diseases in the baby's body, especially in Third Trimester. The dense, lower energies give rise to IUGR, oligohydranmios of various degrees, bleeding issues, reduced fetal movements and so much more.

Second Trimester is a point of balance between mental, emotional and physical manifestation of energies. A well sailed, emotionally strong, calm, peaceful and secure Second Trimester not lays a smooth foundation for the incoming Third Trimester, but also forms the basis of a secure, uneventful birth procedure.

Energy flows to where the concentration goes.

What you think about, you bring about.

THE THIRD TRIMESTER

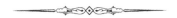

7TH, 8TH, 9TH Months

KEEP CALM, IT IS ONLY BRAXION HICKS.

Some humour needed!

You deserve a medal for making it through another week without stabbing someone with a fork! Your journey of adventure, anticipation, adrenaline, dopamine and serotonin rush is now arriving to a marvelous culmination.

28th week onwards, the dreams, imaginations and the fantasies of having your baby in your arms are taking shape into a near reality. Probably, you have had an experience of visualizing your baby 3D, or 4D at sonography. My all-time favorite connection is 'energetic visualization', where you not only visualize your baby, but also feel as if you are carrying it in your arms. The emotions exchanged are blissful, which no words can explain.

Probably, there is a pattern of your baby's rhythm of life inside you, which you have identified with. A choice has already been made by your unborn, a selection and pattern has already been adapted to an extent.

Reflect back and write down all your feelings and emotions that you've been through at the time of conception, during the First and the Second trimesters.

Why not this marvel of emotion? Just have a sample:

"I am not alone"

Running errands and talking on the phone,

I am pleasantly reminded that I am not alone.

Little tiny hands, a precious rounded knee.

Pushing and twisting that no one can see.

Oh, sweet child kicking up your heels.

It is our little secret that only I can feel.

I look forward to your birth,

When I can kiss your skin,

But for now I will just smile

As I feel you play within.

- Unknown

MAKE YOUR BLUEPRINT JOURNAL

It is delightful if you have been imprinting your baby with awareness right from the very beginning. But if you've just come across this book, or you've been lazy reading and following it for any reason, I would strongly recommended to you the following exercise:

LIFE'S STORY, AT THE TIME OF CONCEPTION: The initial 1-2 months into your pregnancy after conception

1) My prominent emotions (3 or more) during the initial couple of months of pregnancy.

_____

_____

_____

_____

2) My prominent beliefs (3 or more)

_____

_____

_____

_____

3) Two major life situations affecting me and their impacts at mental, emotional and physical levels, if any.

_____

_____

_____

_____

LIFE'S STORY DURING THE FIRST TRIMESTER

1) My prominent emotions (3 or more)

_____

_____

_____

_____

2) My Prominent beliefs (3 or more)

_____

_____

_____

_____

3) Two major life situations affecting me right then-and-their effects.

_____

_____

_____

_____

LIFE'S STORY DURING THE SECOND TRIMESTER

1) My prominent emotions (3 or more).

_____

_____

_____

_____

2) My prominent beliefs (3 or more)

_____

_____

_____

_____

3) Two major life situations affecting me right then-and-their effects.

_____

_____

_____

_____

You have 9 or more major emotions from the time of conception until now. Now write 3 - 4 major ones, repeating ones,

Let me explain this with an example,

At the time of conception, if the major emotions that you experienced were:

Emotions

1. Love
2. Insecurity
3. Fear
4. Courage

Your prominent beliefs were

1. We have financial instability
2. My relationship with my in-laws is burdening
3. My husband doesn't support me enough
4. Our life is beautiful, we are so full of love.

Life situations and their effects

1. Your husband has got a promotion and he is away from you (insecurity).
2. You have performed brilliantly and your involvement at work is more than ever (burden, yet excitement).
3. Someone has been added to your family or gone away (stress of adjustment).
4. You've just shifted to your dream home or have bought a new vehicle (happiness, joy).

Similarly, write down all your emotions and experiences during the time of conception, First and Second Trimester.

Now pick out the most repeating emotions (2 from each category of emotions, beliefs and life's situations).

With this, you exactly know what you have blueprinted your unborn with. These are 30% of the subconscious belief patterns that the mind of your unborn is filled with, already!

It comes to something like this:

1. Insecurity
2. Fear and doubt
3. Love

The child is conditioned to feel and express love, but may turn out to be insecure at the basic level, may have fear of acceptance in future.

Your intuition will guide you and you would exactly know the patterns of beliefs taking shape inside your unborn's mind.

Is it, then, possible to reverse these imprints?

I'd say 100% ,YES ☺ with awareness, though.

Awareness and truth are the two basic components for changing and transforming the belief pattern and conditioning.

When you are in complete awareness and have embraced your truths, all the darkness, all your pitfalls, all your negative beliefs are dissolved.

Embracing the most common fear, the fear of judgement and fear of rejection will lead you to the path of courage and your inner wisdom and light. Real freedom is setting yourself free of your own judgements of right, wrong, beautiful, ugly, slim, fat, rejection and acceptance. When you accept, all that **"is"**, without any complaint, blame, inhibition and fear, is when you fly high in ecstasy of self-realization and your connection with yourself and your baby goes to another level.

Some of you might perceive increased or decreased fetal movements. We have guidelines on the number of fetal movements, which are in optimum range. There are no rules and your baby is 'NOT' under martial surveillance. There is a comfort zone for your unborn, whether the baby is kinesthetic or observing silently, will also determine his intra-uterine movements. You will also know the moods and pattern of your baby's movements. A NO movement for > 6 hrs, definitely calls for a fetal heart beat check-up. If your baby has been active and suddenly goes sluggish, you know, you need to see your doctor..

> *"This is an infinite potential, the human developing inside you is extraordinary."*

By now, you have gained some 6 inches at your waist, the tummy is nicely bulged, your feet and hands are smelted, face puffin, you feel tired and breathless and you have mood swings. You love and hate simultaneously. There is so much chaos; still there is everything in perfect hormony.

And there is an enormous encoded message for all of us, NOW.

You embrace to evolve, become more aware and conscious in your day-to-day *beingness,* by the time you are full of light, you have established the true connection from within and without. This is so truly experienced through pregnancy and just before the baby is to come, there is super chaos. The Third Trimester seems to be full of confusion, heaviness, burden, complaints, excitement, blame, love, ecstasy, fear, doubt, courage, all polarities that your mind can comprehend. And when the "D"-day arrives, all that connect goes for your journey to enlightenment. Also, all the confusion, heaviness, burden, polarities arise before they all merge into one - nothing OR everything. Nothing is when you have become one with all that "is". Everything is when you still choose to view everything as separate.

> **"Clearly, the pregnancy is the path of evolution and the unborn is our GURU."**

The diseases of the Third Trimester like oligohydramnios, polyhydramnios, anhydramnios, IUGR, vaginal bleeding, Pregnancy Induced Hypertension (PIH), gestational, diabetes mellitus (GDM) are all indications of your own thought forms and energy deficits, which can be easily seen in your aura and electromagnetic field before they actually manifest into your physical body and then into your unborn's physical system.

A detailed description of Third Trimester diseases, their causes and possible remedies, will be discussed in my **forthcoming book.**

For now, I cannot stress enough, appealing and requesting you to acknowledge yourself as the 'all-power mother' and do a reality check on your existing thought forms and emotions. A correction now will do a million good to your incoming baby, not only to its physical bodily health, but also could potentially prevent any nursery treatments or admissions. This also does loads of good, in making him/ her mentally and emotionally well-balanced, calm, loving, peaceful and courageous.

"LOVE CURES ALL."

When I say love, I mean 'Self Love'. You can share only what you have for yourself. When you love youself completely, all you can give is ONLY complete love..

Table of diet schedule in the Third Trimester:

This is a general guideline, you will know what to choose and pick.

You need plenty of **energy** in the Third Trimester.

Vitamin K helps your blood to clot, which is important for birth.

Tip: You need 500 kilojoules a day more in the Third Trimester than the Second Trimester, so make sure you have some healthy snacks!

MONDAY

BREAKFAST	SNACK	LUNCH	SNACK	DINNER
Porridge made with milk flavoured with a pinch of cinnamon and a tbsp apple puree Apple juice	Small roll with peanut butter	Couscous cheese salad with pine nuts and currants Fruit custard	Carrot sticks with hummus	Smoked mackerel and spinach pasta

TUESDAY

BREAKFAST	SNACK	LUNCH	SNACK	DINNER
Pot of plain fromage frais mixed with chopped fresh fruit (mango, peach or nectarine) and a tbsp of flaked almonds served on scotch pancakes Berry smoothie	Muffin with a slice of edam	Roast beef and rocket on a wholegrain Baguette Small bunch of grapes	Thick slice of banana bread	Creamy chickpea curry

WEDNESDAY

BREAKFAST	SNACK	LUNCH	SNACK	DINNER
Wheat bisk cereal with semi-skimmed with mashed/ sliced banana apple juice	Melon with blueberries and yoghurt	Beetroot soup melon	2 rye crackers with sardine paste	vegetable risotto

THURSDAY

BREAKFAST	SNACK	LUNCH	SNACK	DINNER
Porridge made with milk flavoured with a tbsp of tinned berries in fruit juice Herbal tea	Slice of fruited malt loaf with spread	Pitta with lamb's lettuce, gruyere and grapes Sliced mango	2-3 mini falafels	Creamy haddock and salmon pie with green beans

FRIDAY

BREAKFAST	SNACK	LUNCH	SNACK	DINNER
Wholegrain toast spread with smooth peanut butter yoghurt drink	2 handfuls of walnuts and dried fruit	Cottage cheese, chapati and green salad chopped apple	Fruity flapjack	Soya chops with sweet potato wedges and mango tout

SATURDAY

BREAKFAST	SNACK	LUNCH	SNACK	DINNER
Pot of Greek yoghurt mixed with tbsp chopped dried fruit (apricots, figs or dates), flaked almonds and tbsp muesli (make the night before and keep in the fridge to soften) Orange juice	Rice pot	Toasted ham and cheese wholemeal sandwich pear	Whole meal toast /chapatti with baked beans	vegetable lasagna made with ragl sauce with a mixed side salad

SUNDAY				
BREAKFAST	**SNACK**	**LUNCH**	**SNACK**	**SNACK**
Scrambled eggs on toasted bread with spread yoghurt drink	Strawberry milkshake	Roast chick peas with roast potatoes, carrots and green beans Sultana rice pudding	Cheese on toast	Spinach and cheese quiche

THE EIGHTH MONTH, BIG REVIEW TIME

Your body is not ruined
You are a tigress, who has earned her stripes.
~Anonymous

Our very Indian thought and, also a worldwide notion, as I reach out to mothers through the globe, is that the eighth month is that of "caution and fear". Do you agree?

While a seventh month delivery (27-29) (pre-term) is considered safe and somewhat okay, the eighth month pre-term is dreaded and most feared. It is often understood that a seventh month born has better chances of survival than has the eighth month born. My own observation is that patients uniformly dread and deal with the 'eighth month terror syndrome' that way. But why? That perhaps is the reason why there is a need for a separate chapter and a special mention.

What Makes It So Dreadful?
Let's go back a little and ask another question: Why nine months in the first place? The duration of the pregnancy for humans could have been less or more. Why nine? And what is so special about the eighth month?

I strongly believe and feel that each number is associated with the planet in solar system it corresponds to. It has its own significance in months and duration of pregnancy. Each month is integrated with the energy of the corresponding number. The prominent qualities of these numbers affect the core vibration related to the corresponding month. (We shall discuss it in the **forthcoming volume**) For now, our focus is going to be on the eighth month in this chapter.

The eighth month is the period between 29th and 33nd week of the gestational age. This is the "window of allowance". As after death, "the soul reviews its entire life time it has lived in the present incarnation, before returning to its plane of choice".... ***Many lives, many masters",*** *by the famous psychiatrist, Dr Brian Weiss, M.D.*

Similarly, this is the time of review by the unborn to decide to leave (complete its life cycle inside the womb) and reincarnate to another life after child birth, or to accomplish a learned lesson of life until the eighth month or less and decide not to come to life and simply go back...

Let me explain this ...Compare your life cycle with that of your unborn. Just as you grow through your life, live through your age in numbers, you change, adjust and transform through experienced, choices, lessons and adaptations. One completes a life's journey until one dies, i.e., when one leaves this particular incarnated life. Similarly, an unborn's lifecycle is full of exponential growth from a two-cell body to a billion-celled baby before birth, which has been nourished, malnourished, nurtured and exposed to contrasting emotions, ranging from the densest vibrations to the lightest, from being weak and wrecked to absolute strength and vigor. Eighth month is the time of review by the consciousness of this super conscious soul. The consciousness of the unborn reviews the lessons, path and experiences. The unborn reviews, especially the evolution and growth of the mother that were to be accepted by her through this pregnancy. The pregnancy would continue to progress unhindered, up to the advanced stages, beyond 36 weeks, provided the mother is evolving as she has to. Let's not lose sight of the fact that your unborn is your spiritual guide.

My experience says that eighth month is also the time when several medical challenges show up, such as, sudden rise in the maternal blood pressure, reduction or an acute increase in the fetal movements. The Colour Doppler studies reveal maximum disturbances and challenges at this time. Sudden reduction in liquor, IUGR sets in mostly at this age of gestation. If the mother is distracted with other issues and agendas, other than her pregnancy and the unborn, not enough focused on her own needs, neglecting her observation and perceptions around this pregnancy, sudden challenges crop up and the alarm bell starts ringing high! Once the alarm rings, it becomes inevitable for the mother, couple and family to review the situation by being entirely focused on the pregnancy. Do the correction and proceed to a bumpy ride towards the ninth month. Etiology of fetal demise (death) remains unknown in 25 to 60% of all cases, others being maternal, fetal and placental causes. (*Article 'Revolution of fetal death', Medscape*). With the support of advanced medical treatments and lab investigations, it has become possible to detect these cases in early stages and offer medical treatment. This has definitely helped in reduction of the number of fetal deaths. But let me ask you a few questions here:

- What about the rise in the complications of the Third Trimester?
- What about the fall in the number of natural vaginal deliveries ?
- What about the number of challenged deliveries that result in caesarean surgeries?
- What about the number of would-be mothers (patients) going to bed rest during and after the eighth month due to some maternal or fetal indication?

We, as medical practitioners, have managed to achieve a reduction in the number of intrauterine deaths(IUDs), but what about the quality of the pregnancy outcomes, the number of complications in the later part of pregnancy? All these are on an alarming rise. The number of difficult childbirths is also abnormally increasing.... WHY?

There is no conclusive and assertive answer to this 'why', though the answer may be found in the bridging month of the eighth month, the month of "**Review by the consciousness of the unborn.**"

The entire course of pregnancy, from the month 0 (point of thought of conception) to the eighth month, is reviewed and the unborn's consciousness decides whether to move ahead and reincarnate to the given set of parents, in the given body or just leave, choosing another set of parents who could be more aligned to its soul's purpose. Or maybe, it was only until now that the experience of the evolution through the pregnancy was meant to be or maybe, it decides to return to the same set of parents only after the desirable vibrational shift (consciously or unconsciously) has occurred during the subsequent conception and pregnancy.

You know it intuitively, and can understand why you are, where you are. All the answers are within you. Receive the messages your baby is giving to you so constantly. If your pregnancy is challenged already, it is time to breathe deep, connect within yourself, perceive all that is in your environment and make necessary changes NOW!! The life definitely is not dense and stagnant, it is full of flow and fluidity. Then, why not adapt to the flow?

You may remind yourself of this:

"I learn, observe, experience and integrate all that I have to, during and through this pregnancy. I allow and accept myself to be an evolved being of love and light."

PREPARING FOR THE BIRTH

Preparation for birth is very simple and requires no preparation at all. All you need is trust and faith that all is going to be very fine , as most of the things will happen without much control. You may completely accept the flow and let go of any expectations out of this delivery. However, nutrition has to be through high calories and high energy at this stage as you prepare yourself for the birth. You may prepare at these major levels:

- Mental
- Emotional
- Spiritual
- Physical

Mental preparation:

> *"Birth is not only about making babies. Birth is about making mothers strong, competent, capable mothers who trust themselves and know their inner strength."*
> *-- Barbara Katz Rathman*

Good, you have not lost your focus, for you know focusing on your goals is the best way to grow up mentally and succeed. Here, your goal is to deliver a healthy baby in the most favourable environment possible.

One big mistake which the couples, especially the mothers, commit at this stage is too much focus on the negative side delivery. Why should we speak to ourselves, *"I hope, I will not have a c – section"*?

Or

"Can I go for a c – section, I can't bear the pain."

Both of these thought forms are definitely no sign of any mental strength. The first is that of DOUBT and the second is that of FEAR. Both will drain your energies. The more you focus on surgical delivery, the more you will attract it. On the other hand, your focus could be on:

- How can I have the most simple, effortless, beautiful and easy experience of delivering this baby?
- How can I bring our baby into this world with love and ease?

You will see a lot changing inside you as your point of view changes. You are no longer focused on how the delivery will happen. Instead, you are more keen on having a healthy baby in the most beautiful and easy way!

Emotional preparation

"Out of suffering have emerged the strongest souls; the most massive characters are scarred with scars."
-- Kahlil Gibran

This is the time to consciously stay at a vibration of courage, love and peace.

When you are at peace and you accept things happening for your highest good, you are being courageous and unconditionally loving.

Say to yourself:

- I give and receive unconditional love.

- I am at peace.

Just repeating and reminding yourself of these two powerful affirmations each day will definitely keep you in high vibrations of love and peace. It is these vibrations that cause magic and miracles to happen.

You can't expect anything beautiful and magical happening to you, when you are filled with fear, doubt or anger.

Stay away from the situations that bring any emotional drama to your life. If you are persistently experiencing them, then ask yourself:

"What is in me that is attracting this emotional drama and story in my life?"

As I have said earlier, awareness is the key to solution. Find out your emotional baggage and sabotages which have attracted these stories in your life.

Spiritual/ energetic preparation

"To be pregnant is to be vitally alive, thoroughly woman, and distressingly inhabited. Soul and spirit are stretched – along with body – making pregnancy a time of transition, growth, and profound beginnings."
-- Anne Christian Buchanan

Spiritual/ energetic preparation is aligning your energies for the most suitable birth. This is the most basic alignment that will get you to emotional and mental alignment. Meditation and breathing exercises are important tools in energetic alignment.

Meditation

Meditation does not mean you have to sit in a secluded or a green place at 4:00 AM--though it is ideal ☺. You can be at your most comfortable and favourite place, seated or lying, anytime of the day. *Brahma muhurata* (the hours before sunrise) is the ideal time, as most of the people are sleeping then, the mass conscious thoughts are much less denser in the environment at the time. You just need to relax your entire body, all your body parts and become aware of only the PRESENT MOMENT. Listen to all the sounds and slowly, as you start focusing on a point inside your mind, these sounds will vanish and you will come to a point of NO THOUGHTS. If the thoughts still persist, say a hello to them, inflate them in a colourful, light-weight balloon and let it rise high in the sky. These thoughts will leave you soon, one by one. This is possible with regular practice. This is the point when all energetic balance takes place inside and outside of you.

You may watch/listen to meditative videos that you most resonate with. (Find them at www.birththenewearth.com and Awakening in Womb (YouTube channel). Visualization and guided meditations are also good for beginners.

Breathing Exercises

Breathing is equivalent to the life force, the *'prana'*. How you breathe has a direct impact on the health and growth of any cell of your body. A full, deep breath results in accelerated growth of the cells in your body at any given moment of time, including the eggs, sperms, the cells and tissues of your tiny growing baby inside you. Count your usual breaths per minute, observe whether these are shallow or deep, and whether they fill up your chest, partially or fully.

A Deep abdominal breathing at 7 to 8 breaths per minute is ideal.

Physical preparation

When you are energetically, emotionally and mentally prepared, physical preparation happens automatically, as each of these ingredients manifests in your physical body and environment. A few rituals which may help you are:

1. Daily morning walks
2. Stretching exercises
3. Butterfly and squatting exercises
4. Kegel's exercises

You will find a number of other exercising rituals and routines. You don't have to undergo them as some forced regime. In fact, you need to pick and choose which you enjoy most. Exercise does not have to be a burden on you, but an enjoyable experience. Diet will play an important role. You may increase your fat and fatty acid intake and have good amount of proteins and carbohydrates. Carbohydrates will keep your energy levels and mental focus high.

> *"Life is a mirror and will reflect back to the thinker what*
> *he thinks into it."*
> *-- Ernest Holmes*

Daily look into the mirror

Look at your entire body from head to toe, appreciate all your body parts and your bulged out tummy, remind yourself that you are unique and special as you are to bring another unique and special soul to this world. Look into your own eyes and send boundless love to yourself by repeating this:

"I love you (your name) more and more and more".

Wearing your happy and dazzling smile every day, all this will prepare you well for your grand day.

It's one wondrous experience to communicate with your unborn, such as:

> *"No one else will ever know the strength of my love for you. After all, you are the only one who knows what my heart sounds like, from inside."*

> *"The power and intensity of your contractions cannot be stronger than you, because they are you."*

> *- Unknown*

PART 3

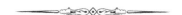

CONSCIOUS BIRTHING

"The history of man for nine months preceding his birth would, probably, be far more interesting and contain events of greater moment, than all the threescore and ten years that follow it."

--Samuel Taylor Coleridge

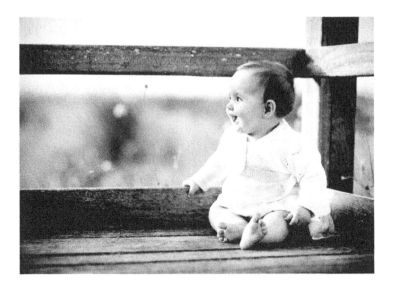

"There are only three events in a man's life: birth, life, and death. He is not conscious of being born, he dies in pain, and he forgets to live.
--Jean De La Bruyere

What is conscious birthing and why is it important and how does it affect our lives? Having assisted delivering more than 10,000 babies, I have studied extensively the correlation between the way a child is brought into this world and the way it affects the child's behaviour in his/her later life. The experience of the process of birthing itself gets deeply marked in the subconscious of the baby, the very first imprints and inferences out of these experiences become permanent trait patterns of this baby.

How can it affect the future life of our just born?

Let us review this with an example. For a moment, just try to be in the shoes of your newborn and try to experience what he or she may feel and experience. (For the convenience, let's refer the newborn as a she here). Imagine, you are asked to take a journey into space to the Planet Mars. You are willing to embark upon the journey, have a fancy well-equipped and an amazing vessel. You have accepted the vessel as your temporary home, after a few initial hiccups, adjustments to the new environment and your new life in the space. Wonderful ! You are imagining with excitement, anticipation and maybe, with a little fear, your life on Mars. But what a joy of this adventurous journey!

The grand-day of the landing is approaching nearer, you are preparing yourself for it—excited! By now, this spacecraft is your comforting home. The throttle of the engine is assuring that the things are functioning fine. You have even started loving your home. You don't know much about the inhabitants of Mars, their existance is a question mark, yet you are looking forward to the rendezvous though! You are securely attached to your mother vessel through a cord, an assuring wire that ensures you not straying, but being around your loving home. The grand day arrives, you are landing! Time to step out, you may be too excited and ready to jump off, or maybe, you just don't wish to, and refuse to come out fearful.., you must, though!

You meet Martians as soon as you are out of your vessel home. Now imagine this: A loving, assuring and a warm pair of hands with comforting and loving emotions hold you, caressing you, repeating the words of comfort and assurance, holding you gently.

You immediately start relaxing and feeling calmer and may even develop some fancy for the people who have received you... You are not afraid, even when your cord is cut and you are separated from your mother vessel, you are secure and look forward to your stay with joy and happy anticipation.

On the other hand imagine this, you are being pushed out of your vessel, being pulled simultaneously, to different, strange voices, faces— some harsh words receive you, you are mechanically passed from one stranger to another, exposed to severe bright, unfamiliar coloured lights on your face, not able to see and focus, not understanding the language, but understanding the feeling of indifference for sure, you are *AFRAID AS HELL!*

You desperately want go back to the comfort of your vessel which by now is impossible. The first basic memory and emotion imprinted deep inside you is that of FEAR and non-belief. This basic memory and the feeling around it form the basic character of your newborn's personality, not to mention the vessel is the mother and the Martians are the people assisting the delivery.

> *"Obviously, there is pain in childbirth. But giving birth is also a moment of awe and wonder, a moment when the true miracle of 'aliveness', and of a woman's amazing part in that miracle, is suddenly experienced in every cell of one's body. It is in that sense truly an altered state of consciousness."*
> *---Rennie Eisler*

Dr David Chamberlain, former President of The Association for Prenatal and Perinatal Psychology and Health (APPPAH), in his book, *'The Mind of Your Newborn Baby'* writes and demonstrates that *"New-borns are cognitive humans with the ability to discriminate and experience the world in sophisticated ways. Not only do they perceive and understand their births, but they can hear, feel, and learn while still in utero."* He further writes :*"Records of birth memory obtained in hypnosis span the last hundred years."* Dr. Otto Rank (**The Trauma of Birth 1924**), another visionary therapist, saw links between birth and many problems. An early *associate of Freud, believed that virtually all psychological problems, if not all human behaviour, could be understood as reactions to trauma at birth.*

"An American analyst, Nandor Foder, viewed birth as an agonizing ordeal for the baby, a transition he compared to dying. He believed birth was so traumatic that we all develop a protective amnesia about it. The real memory is preserved in the unconscious mind and he believed that it emerges in dreams and behaviour". In 1970, psychologist Arthur Janov believed that early hurts in life were foundation of most mental problems.

So, what is conscious birthing?

Conscious birthing is the delivery of the baby through the process of normal birthing or a C- section, but with a complete awareness. It primarily constitutes three parts:

- The period, when the mother is in labour
- The period, of the birthing process, i.e., delivery of the baby.
- The period of immediately post-natal care, i.e, immediately after birth

During the time, when the mother is perceiving labour pain or she is preparing herself for a c- section, there are a variety of emotions that she undergoes. It is of reliance and significance to understand that all these emotions she undergoes right then, are actually sedimenting deep inside the subconscious, the deeper layers of the new-born's mind. These emotions are transferred from the mother to the baby, 'as-in' forming it's basic mindset, which shows up as the baby progresses on it's journey to infancy, toddlerhood, adolescence and adulthood. Mother has to be conscious while bearing down the pain. Is she being courageous, is she passing on her love, is she being thankful, full of gratitude? Or, is she complaining, regretting even blaming? Whatever may her feelings be, every single of them is being transmuted to her child. Even we, as doctors or midwives, cannot receive the baby mechanically, like some product popping out of a sophisticated machine. The baby is braving out of the birthing canal, a bit fearful, anxious, maybe, excited.. How do you receive a guest from a foreign country, visiting your country for the first time? Yes, you got it right ! We too, as doctors or midwives may receive the baby with full awareness, love, care, sensitivity and positivity, by reassuringly saying aloud, " *Baby, you have come into this beautiful world, you are very secure, you are being loved*". And with the same gentleness and sensitivity, the child may be put to the mother and she, passing all her love, comfort and assuring emotions, which actively build the psyche of the newborn. (The neuron connection is now happening at an electrifying pace) Thus, the child becomes (or not) loving, secure, caring, flowing with life, accepting life with courage, vis-avis when the baby is pulled out mechanically, put somewhere in the receiving trolley, multiple hands and voices handling him, the baby is fearful, in doubt and suspecting people! He has tendencies of asking questions such as : **why am I here? I** don't want to be here. Who are these people? The baby is already insecure. Fear, doubt and insecurity are it's first emotions! So, it totally depends upon the mother, the way she delivers and upon us, the birth assisting people, the way we handle the birth, that the baby gets the first sense of security and assurance of calmness and peace.

Dr Thomas Verny, in his book, **"The Secret Life of the Unborn child'** writes, "How he is born-- whether it is painful or easy, smooth or violent-- largely determines who he becomes and how he will view the world around him. Whether he is five, ten, forty or seventy, a part of him always looks out at the world through the eyes of the newly born child he once was."

Dr Chamberlain has some very interesting observations in his book, in which he writes, "a person born prematurely acts differently in the same situation than a person who was born late. Unwanted children may invite rejection, those breech-born may go at relationship backwards, the caesarean-born have trouble completing things and incubator babies may grow up acting as if they are separated from love by a glass wall, apart from being non-trusting and fearful."

So,

How to prepare yourself for birthing?

One is Physical and another way is Emotional, mental.

Physical preparation,
You all know. You are very well guided by your family, doctor and the hospital. Your test reports, ultrasound, colour Doppler tests, the doctor's prescription file, your and your baby's pre-and-post-labour kit and a few things more, are all very good. Thus, the planning and preparation, both are satisfactory.

What about the second aspect?

I find so many youngsters, first-time mothers, approaching me and my colleagues for elective cesarean births. There is an alarming rise in the incidence of cesarean sections. A significant number of would-be moms don't want to undergo this pain. So, they choose the easier, shortcut path deciding for an elective surgery. This issue needs to be addressed to, yet again, as it plays a profoundly important role in the child's future development. The natural procedure of birthing is not something random. It has been specifically designed by God Himself. Indeed, the natural birthing process is the best option, unless there is an absolute indication for a caesarean section. The last thing you would want your child to remember, feel and believe is that her/his mother was not courageous enough to face the pain of natural birth. This doesn't end here, this attitude of not being able to face the life's challenges and difficulties and running away from situations may become the character of your newborn and the future adult !

Why is it important?

The emotional part of the birthing is what you undergo. However, the normal procedure of birthing is constantly reminding you of certain values, which are very integral to motherhood.

Patience, courage, surrender, belief and faith

With faith, you completely surrender. You develop the patience and the courage to undergo the experience. You say "YES", I am there, I will undergo this experience and then you talk to your child, emotionally and mentally, *"look baby, I am winning, you are winning too; let's do it together!"* Your child undergoes the process of birthing, while passing through the birth canal, he/she is exposed to harsh challenges, such as, pressure of the narrow, squeezing birth canal. The baby is time and again reminded to be courageous, to face it, to surrender, to have faith, to believe that everything is going to be good. This is the first challenge which your child shall face and come out a warrior!!

Now just imagine, when you go to a doctor asking her for caesarean section, unwilling to undergo the natural procedure of birthing with some excuses, what are you telling your child? Your mom is not courageous, she can't face it. She does not have enough faith and belief in herself and her delivering team. She is not willing to surrender. And when you communicate this to your unborn, at the subconscious level, what do you think is going to happen to him/her? This is one solid programming which we do to our children when we avoid normal birthing procedure for the shortcut of a surgical birth. There is no denying there could be absolute and relative indications for a C - section, but otherwise deliberately resolving to escape the normal birth pain shows a less motherly, loving emotion. Fear diminishes LOVE !!

Really !

Believe, it is not at all worth it !

Apart from this, when we go for a caesarean section directly without any indication, we are also knowingly taking the child away from the immunity that he/she is going to acquire while passing through the birth canal. A lot of immune system is initiated here. So, young girls, first time or the second time mothers, please go for the natural birthing procedure as much as possible. It is integrated to you and your child's evolution. After undergoing this entire procedure, you evolve to the next level of patience, courage, stamina and surrender and when you have done it, your child comes out a warrior, much like you!

PART 4

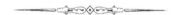

CONSCIOUS PARENTING

"Children are educated by what the grown-up is and not by his talk."

- Carl Jung

CONSCIOUS PARENTING

High Pace : Changing Gears Of Power In The First Year Of
Infancy.
"Your child's spirit is infinitely wise."
-- Dr Tsabary

But how does your child wake you up ?
To connect with your child, you first need to be connected to yourself. Despite our best intentions, we enslave our children to the emotional inheritance that we received from our parents, binding them to the legacy of our ancestral past. A certain child enters our life with its individual love, courage, troubles, difficulties, challenges and stubbornness, in order to help us become aware of how much we have yet to grow. Each child has a pace that it will move and catch on to.

In our case, both our children, Pranicka and Arjun, are starkly different.

When our daughter was born, I was working very hard, almost 12 hours a day, in a government hospital labour room set-up. The number of deliveries happening per 24 hours then was anywhere between 70 to 90 per day.

How the system worked and how we managed falls as a nightmare to me now. I was overworked, hardly paying any attention to myself or my baby's needs during my first pregnancy. My food habits were erratic and off schedule mostly. It was not until the 29th week that I was advised by a senior, "If you are to have a live baby, you better quit and take some rest. This all (work) would go endlessly anyways." The next thing I remember today is I had quit my job then and there.

My sonogram showed an average-sized baby, with markedly reduced water. I was frightened and full of fear. I was drained mentally and emotionally. We still lived in a post-graduate, government hostel accommodation, as my husband Dr Pradeep was pursuing his post-graduate degree then.

All the bed rest and nutrition at a late 30th week could not see me through, and I was scared and insecure. It goes without saying that I landed in a caesarean and Pranicka in the nursery for a good period of 8 hours. Although healthy, she needed to be kept under observation. Precious golden moments away from us! (I was clueless about the graph of blueprinting back then!)

My perspectives of life completely transformed, as I held my daughter in my arms. I decided to quit working completely and be the mom for Pranicka 24x7. I was just that for another good 17 months. All my identities, those of being a doctor, wife, daughter-in-law and a daughter, got completely dissolved and all I could be was a mother.

My fears and insecurities washed away and I flew high on hope. Pranicka's milestones were way ahead. She was standing and walking at nine months. She was sharp, observant and intelligent, very playful, a happy, smiling and an attractive baby. As she went to her playschool, she was seen as bright and participating. We, of course, were very proud parents.

My own psyche during the months I carried her, was to be ahead of time at all my tasks, complete all the work ASAP, and then get on to another. Pranicka had the same character early at everything-- talking, walking, running and dancing.

We became over-expecting parents as we believed she was immensely gifted.

As she was entering her third year, we wanted to have another baby and have the family completed early. This time, I was conscious not to rush into things. I adapted a laid-back lifestyle. I was working in day time, in a not-so-demanding private practice from 9 to 2 pm only. But my food intake and exercise regimen were both ideally on course.

My weight gain was enormous, almost 20 kg, had a very healthy, good-sized baby. The entire pregnancy was uneventful and happy.

This pregnancy was also landing in a c–section, as my previous scar was thinning and my labour was not improving. We decided to get our second baby delivered at a hospital run by my friend. My husband, a pediatrician, was to be our baby's doctor. As soon as Arjun came out into this world, he landed in the hands of his father, in secure, warm and a loving pair of hands!

Arjun had his milestones delayed, was late to walk and very late to talk. He was a quiet and not so social baby. He would cry at the mention of playschool and never wanted to go out anywhere, ever.

His writing and reading skills were delayed too, in contrast to those of our daughter, who had the ability to identify the alphabets at an early age of 15 months. (We never taught her, she self-learned through the teachers organ game that she received as a gift on her first birthday!) She talked and wrote at one plus of age. Here, we did the same big mistake that most parents do. We kept comparing Arjun with his sister, repeatedly humming that Arjun was a noticeable laggard against Pranicka and was not matching her brilliant quotients.

A couple of years down the lane, the situation persisted and our frustration started growing. We simply thought that we could not parent both our children the same way. In the process, we forgot that the two were different individuals, who had different personalities. After this realization, we decided to give the power to our kids by giving them options to make their own choices and shine in their respective lights.

We freed them to make independent choices, of course, under close supervision--right from food, clothing to their style of education and learning. As a result, they understood very early on that marks and grades, albeit significant and indicative, were merely the systems that the schools had adopted to quantitatively analyze the knowledge the kids had. We, too as parents, shifted our gears of thinking and became less interested in their grades or ranks at school. We would have discussions around the subjects and everyone was free to voice his/her opinion. We just inspired the kids to dream big and pursue their passions. Our place had become a centre of great resonance where inspiration, free will, dreaming potential flourished and positive thinking ruled the roost. In the obtaining environment, Arjun started blossoming. He got admission through a national-level entrance exam at one of India's leading boarding schools, WELHAM BOYS' SCHOOL, DEHRADUN, nestled in the valley of Dehradun. A non-achiever had transformed into an achiever and an inspiring child. He is now a 'consistent scholar' at school and a level 'A' swimmer, representing his school at various national-level events.

Our dear family friend and a well-wisher Rachna Goel, from Hyderabad, once remarked, "Pranicka and her mom give serious relationship goals to people. They have a lovely relationship and are blessed to have each other." Thank you Rachna, for your kind words, we are still on the road to learning and moving ahead.

My journey as a parent so far has taught me a lot, I am still learning and have a very long way to go. A few of my learnings I wish to share with you:

- You must have faith, trust and belief as core value between yourself and your child (you must trust your child, as much as you trust yourself).
- Your child's behaviour mainly reflects your own conduct, most of the time. Who in the family is your child reflecting? This could be the guidance and also a source of remedy.
- The best that you can do to your child is: Keep your own conditionings, belief patterns away! Your child's light is enough for her/him to shine.
- Your child in her 1st year after birth loves these three things the most--exploring, exploring and exploring. Your house and this world in general is a vast learning ground for her. What we assume to be her 'playing' is her exploring, learning and understanding of the world around her.
- Listen to your child, pay attention to her/his actions. This divine guidance in your life needs respect.
- Even as a newborn, she craves for some privacy and space. Please do not showcase your babies as some "won trophies".
- Do not rush to assist and lend a helping hand to your child at one go, give her room, space and time to learn from her own mistakes. But observe that she is not exposed to danger. If she falls down, let her experience the pain and 'victory' of getting up on her own, and then when she stands up, pat her back.
- If possible, omit the words, like, "cannot", "do not", "never", from your conversation with your child. Remember, you

are your child's heroine and she will adapt to everything without questioning you ever. So, when it is a "you can NEVER" she believes "she can never", and when It is "you are brave, you can do it", it is that she is brave and can do it. It is this simple!

- Hugs, gentle pats and words of motivation may be handy and inspiring and you should be generous at showering them.
- Always remember, your child is not your personal private property. She is an eternal being with her own personality and life plan. Please, do not over-indulge with your kids, offer them choices and the liberty to take decisions.

"THE RISK OF LABELLING IS THAT IT CHANGES THE WAY
WE PERCEIVE THINGS."
- JENNIFER EBERHARDT, social psychologist

Adaptation from the book, **Soul Song**, by my dear friend, a highly evolved soul, Mana:

"The kids are here on Earth with a purpose and require specific methods to adjust their beingness to the family's, parents' and the society's vibrations. When diagnosed with an "abnormal mental inclination", such as ADS (attention deficit syndrome), hyperactivity, or low attention span, children and adults, who become nervously distressed in loud and chaotic environments are diagnosed as abnormal and labeled abnormal in our society's norms as the reference point. The definition of 'normal' and 'correct' is very relative and should be considered at individual non-discriminating manner. For example: The child, Ishan in the Bollywood film, *Taare Zameen Par* (2007) was labeled autistic. The movie was released by Disney as *"Stars on Earth"* (2007) and showcases the special abilities and issues that children diagnosed with autism sometimes face.

"Some new age filmmakers are devoted to presenting another aspect of the illness versus progress debate. They are proposing that whatever is happening - is a gift.

"New age children may also include many labeled as dyslexic. A child who doesn't speak or write until a later stage of development may be communicating in another way. The ability to use all of the brain, and tap into the vastness of soul space via the right brain would logically lead to differences in speaking and writing abilities.

"If these children are not fitting into the system, then maybe, the family and schooling systems need to understand the greater picture. New age souls have come with the development of new traits and intelligences, a definite idealism, artistic ability, and the ability to experience the **"multi-verse"** as multiple dimensions of existence.

"One thing is certain: these new age children, the highly evolved souls are coming as a great gift to progress of the planet. We are meant to learn from them and grow with them. Systems are meant to change from competitive to cooperative, fearful to loving, autocratic and controlling to diplomatic and fair, as we all come to a better understanding of who we are as immensely powerful interconnected beings of Spirit.

"It is important to know that some infants are unique. It is, however, counterproductive to label them as mentally ill and commence to train them to fit into the "majority", or the accepted norm.

"We could just as easily label them as highly evolved beings, and train everyone else to be more like them. Maybe, there is a way to encourage them and collectively gain from their creative and multi-dimensional abilities.

"It is commonly known that hyperactivity and attention deficits also arise from food allergies and sensitivity to gluten and food colouring. One study in the USA found that 60% of hyperactive children were eventually cured of ADHD or ADD when they discovered their food allergies and corrected their diet.

"Other children have responded well to Bach flower and homeopathic remedies which harmonize the vibration of the body. It may be that the high bodily vibration of some new age children has trouble adjusting to the specific vibrations of certain foods and artificial food ingredients. One must independently research as this information is largely suppressed by the industry.

"One may also work with mantra, soothing classical music and massage with natural, aromatic oils. Those are treatments which work to harmonize the high bodily vibration of new age children and may be effective in "grounding them" to Earth's vibration."

On the side of MANA's life-changing observations, I would also like you to understand that you the mother or the father know what is best for your child, or better still, know that your child is guiding you. There is no cut out "best" method of parenting. Every method is the best method which allows your baby, an infant or your child, to bloom and blossom, weaving you and your child happily in a joyous relationship. A mother for sure, intuitively knows what her child's best faculties are and what is not so exciting to the child. Please always listen to your own intuition, your sixth sense, and never ever overrule or ignore your child's opinion. Her sentences, vocabulary and dialogue delivery may be kiddish and childlike (of course!), but always remember, she carries the wisdom of the source within herself.

I further suggest that life is not to be taken seriously. We are to observe and learn through the choices that we make, really we don't have time to judge or blame, there is so much to choose from and create our own lives. The beauty is that we have the power to change and transform within us if only we looked and went inside of ourselves, we would find all the answers. For now, all beloved mothers and fathers, just become aware of this infinite power of choices that you have and choose wisely, let loose, have fun , enjoy yourself and have beautiful lives. To have faith is like being that magic wand yourself that you want to hold in your hands. Do not think too much, just allow the faith and energy to work its way, because it works when you ALLOW it to.

Another thing, never forget to count your blessings. You need to realize that what you have is what some people may be dreaming to have right this very moment. With gratitude open the new doors of expansions and abundance. Abundance of joy and happiness, abundance of laughter and blessings in your life, all shall fall in place.

Wish you a happy pregnancy, birthing and an ever joyful parenting.

SOURCES AND READINGS

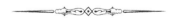

- THE BIOLOGY OF BELIEF, *by Dr Bruce H. Lipton.*
- THE SECRET LIFE OF YOUR UNBORN CHILD *by Dr Thomas R. Verney, John Kelly.*
- THE MIND OF YOUR NEWBORN BABY *by Dr David Chemberlain*
- YOU CAN HEAL YOUR LIFE *by Louise Hay*
- YOU CAN HEAL YOUR BODY *by Louise Hay*
- SECRETS OF MILLIONAIRE MIND *by T. Harv Eker.*
- *SOUL SONG, by Mana*
- THE AWEKENING : 9 PRINCIPLES FOR FINDING THE COURAGE TO CHANGE YOUR *LIFE by Sidra Jafri*
- CONVERSATIONS WITH GOD(all 3 parts) *by Neale Donald Walsch*
- THE HONEYMOON EFFECT *by Dr Bruce H. Lipton*

SHARE THE WISDOM

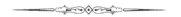

"The mark of true wealth is determined by how much one can give away." - T .Harv Eker

This book teaches you to observe your thought forms and to challenge your limiting unserving belief patterns, habits and rituals with regard to your life as a would-be parent.

The goal of this book has been to assist you in your evolution, become aware and raise your consciousness to be able to attract that highly-evolved soul in your life, as your child. Raising consciousness by observing your limiting habits and by taking massive actions on the basis of your choices rather than acting on the basis of programming from the past, hence blueprinting the subconscious mind of your unborn for its highest good.

By now, you have realized that the true essence of transformation starts with "self" at the same time not all "about" self. As you discover your light and empower yourself, you are transforming the two of you. Imagine what may happen when this entire new incoming generation is consciously conceived, carried, birthed and parented? What will be the future of humanity like? What could be the future of this planet?

Be the light to enlighten hundreds and thousands of others.

I, therefore, ask you to share this message of evolution, consciousness and empowerment with others. Get the message of this book out to as many people as possible. Commit to letting many of your friends, who are in the family way or are parents already, know about it or consider getting it for them as life-changing gift. Become the channel of the divine by helping them raise their consciousness and hence, the consciousness of the planet.

THANK YOU

Inspired by T. Harv Eker's incredible tips in the book, **Secrets Of The Millionaire Mind**

ACKNOWLEDGEMENTS

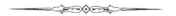

We generally are trapped in our lives with the feelings of "If this goes well, all goes well". My journey of transformation began with the realization," When I go well, all goes well".

During this time of great personal transformation, I am blessed and guided by both spiritual and incarnated forces. I am indebted to the Spirits of Masters, for I am fully aware that these are the forces that have guided me in bringing this message across. I feel Sai Baba ji's overflowing radiance and grace all around me, as I remain constantly guided in the realm of divine ecstasy.

I wish to make special mention of Dr. Bruce H Lipton, whose 'Biology of Belief' came in through, just when it was needed.

My deepest gratitude to all the divine souls of unborns and newborns, whom I got connected with, who revealed so much 'of here' and 'beyond'. Thank you, thousands of mothers, expecting parents, for opening up and pouring your hearts and allowing for the healing to flow. Thanks to all the patients for showing up for a session, just when I needed a healing and a de-layering on my ownself.

Thanks to all my teachers and guides for numerous workshops, seminars and sessions that I have attended. I am who I am, because of your contribution in my growth. Gratitude!

My soul buddies, dear friends and family. All of you have contributed to my being of who I am today. Love you all! You know, I am writing about you here.

Blessings and thanks to you, Mahi, Rose Verma and Manish Punetha for the inputs, editing efforts and illustrations.

My Journalist dad, Mr. S .P. Singh, for believing in the concepts of this book, believing in me and guiding with his knowledge in this humble effort. If not for him , this book would not see the light of the day. My mom, Mrs. Poonam Singh, who has been my pillar of strength always and without whose inspiration, I would not have been what I am today! Your pure, unconditional love and dedication as parents have been the light on my path. Love you, dad and mom!

Our children, Pranicka and Arjun, for helping me discover "my own self". My world begins with you, my lifelines!

This acknowledgement would not be complete without a special thank you to Dr. Pradeep Chauhan, my husband, the love of my life, my eternal soulmate. I am ....because you are.

MIRACLE MEDICAL MISSIONS'S AWAKENING IN WOMB EVENTS

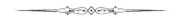

'Awakening in Womb' (AIW) empowering seminars and workshops. Online 'hand-holding' programmes on 'Blueprinting The Subconscious Mind Of Your Unborn'

- AIW, Four hours FREE workshop for aspiring to be parent couples, pregnant mothers, Couples with fertility challenges, parents of the new-borns.
- AIW 2 Days intensive workshop for couples aspiring to be parents, pregnant mothers, couples challenged with fertility issues, parents of the new born.
- AIW, 1 Day Foundation course for all categories.
- AIW, Conscious Pregnancy, the 9 months hand- holding ,mentorship programme.
- First Trimester hand-holding programme .
- Second Trimester hand-holding programme,
- Third Trimester hand-holding programme.
- AIW, 'Conceive the Miracle' (CTM)
- AIW, Cosmic Fertility (CF)
- AIW, Power Parenting Programme (PPP)
- Online AIW Webinars, Tutorials, Sessions.

Details at, www.birththenewearth.com

Facebook Page : Awakening In Womb

YouTube Channel : Awakening In Womb.

Email : info@birththenewearth.com

Phone No. : +91-800-615-6664

             : +91-800-615-6669

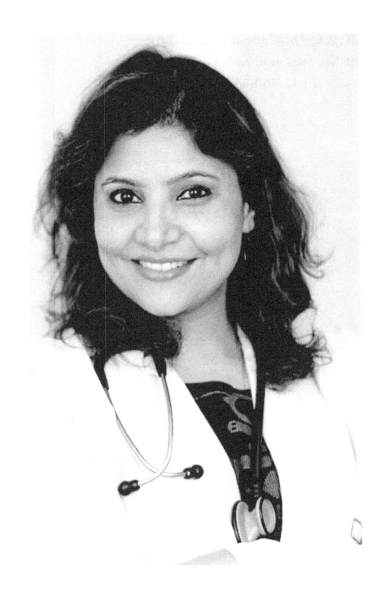

MEET DR MONIKA SINGH

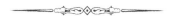

Dr Monika Singh, as an ardent student of life, remains in hot pursuit of miracles. Having experienced the magical powers of subconscious mind and belief programming early on in her life, she found herself both "intrigued and freed" as she carved her path into the understanding of deeper layers of subconscious mind, belief patterns and conditionings. She experienced her life unfolding and decoding itself proportionally to the subconscious mind programmes existing in her own mind. She found that this was universally true for every single living human being. This led to an extensive research, learning, acquiring knowledge and applying it to greater good of the masses.

Dr Monika has extensively applied her knowledge from her experiences and the research work she has carried out on her patients and clients over the last seven years. She has formulated applicable tools, techniques and processes, used them for her patients, would-be couples and pregnant women, empowering them to be of immense use by themselves, primarily on the subject of **'Blueprint The Subconscious Of Your Unborn'.** The number of these patients and clients has run into over a 1,000 now ! And she has come across some incredibly miraculous results!

Dr Monika is on a mission to integrate ancient spiritual birthing wisdom and techniques with modern scientific methods of obstetric care and birthing. She is an '**Awakening Facilitator At**

Womb', Sonologist, practitioner of Obstetrics, Speaker & an internationally published author of the books, '**The Miracle Mission'** and '**Awakening In Womb'.**

Dr Monika's Vision: To be a catalyst in building a tribe of aligned individuals, to help unleash the power that parents possess to attract the kind of souls they wish to, as their kids. Help expecting mothers not only to cruise with ease, confidence and conviction through the trying challenges of pregnancy, but also to empower them with tools to identify and blueprint the desired, high-vibration souls as their babies.

Currently running a multi-speciality Hospital, alongside her Pediatrician husband, Dr Pradeep Chauhan, they shifted their base, 9 years ago, from a high-profile hospital practice in Delhi to a deep, back-water interior, with the intention to serve rural population.

Dr Monika is actively involved in educating the expecting parents, fertility seekers, and parents of the newborns. Her patients with infertility issues, pregnancy-related challenges, birthing and parenting concerns of infancy have especially benefited from her research-based services. Practicing Obstetrician for nearly two decades now, she has on her scroll of toil a large number of walking, talking "**Miracle Babies''.**

Transformational workshops, sessions and classes are regularly held under Dr Monika's '**Miracle Medical Mission'** Programme. Thousands of expecting parents, patients with pregnancy-related challenges, couples aspiring to be blessed with babies have benefited from these programmes. The life-changing interactions and scientific-spiritual techniques, not only to help the parents move forward in life, but also to provide a platform of neutrality for the babies to come. Dr Monika welcomes you all, looking for respite from the issues and challenges that she raises in this book. See you soon , sometime!

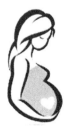

NOTES

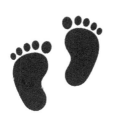

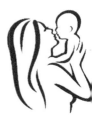